HUMAN TRAFFICKING

A Treatment Guide for Mental Health Professionals

HUMAN TRAFFICKING

A Treatment Guide for
Mental Health Professionals

Edited by

John H. Coverdale, M.D., Ed.D.
Mollie R. Gordon, M.D.
Phuong T. Nguyen, Ph.D.

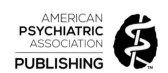

AMERICAN
PSYCHIATRIC
ASSOCIATION
PUBLISHING

If you wish to buy 50 or more copies of the same title, please go to www.appi.org/specialdiscounts for more information.

Copyright © 2020 American Psychiatric Association Publishing
ALL RIGHTS RESERVED
First Edition

Manufactured in the United States of America on acid-free paper
24   23   22   21   20   5   4   3   2   1

American Psychiatric Association Publishing
800 Maine Avenue SW
Suite 900
Washington, DC 20024-2812
www.appi.org

Library of Congress Cataloging-in-Publication Data
Names: Coverdale, John H., editor. | Gordon, Mollie R., editor. | Nguyen, Phuong T., editor.
Title: Human trafficking : a treatment guide for mental health professionals / edited by, John H. Coverdale, Mollie R. Gordon, Phuong T. Nguyen.
Other titles: Human trafficking (Coverdale)
Description: First edition. | Washington, DC : American Psychiatric Association Publishing, [2020] | Includes bibliographical references and index.
Identifiers: LCCN 2020019080 (print) | LCCN 2020019081 (ebook) | ISBN 9781615372485 (paperback ; alk. paper) | ISBN 9781615373154 (ebook)
Subjects: MESH: Human Trafficking—psychology | Psychological Trauma—therapy | Crime Victims—psychology | United States
Classification: LCC HQ281 (print) | LCC HQ281 (ebook) | NLM WM 172.5 | DDC 364.15/51—dc23
LC record available at https://lccn.loc.gov/2020019080
LC ebook record available at https://lccn.loc.gov/2020019081

British Library Cataloguing in Publication Data
A CIP record is available from the British Library.

Contents

About the Editors ix

Contributors xi

Preface xv
    John H. Coverdale, M.B. Ch.B., M.D.,
      M.Ed., FRANZCP
    Mollie R. Gordon, M.D.
    Phuong T. Nguyen, Ph.D.

1 Becoming a Trafficked Person 1
    Ronald Chambers, M.D., FAAFP

2 Epidemiology of Human Trafficking:
COMPLEXITIES AND INTERSECTIONS OF
VULNERABILITY, RISK, AND EXPLOITATION 19
    Melissa I.M. Torres, Ph.D., M.S.W.

3 By the Right Name: WHAT DOES IT ACTUALLY
MEAN TO "SCREEN" AND "ASSESS" FOR
TRAFFICKING IN HEALTH CARE? 31
    Makini Chisolm-Straker, M.D., M.P.H.

4 Barriers to Identification of Trafficked
Persons in Health Care Settings 49
Frances Recknor, L.C.S.W., Dr.P.H.
Hanni Stoklosa, M.D., M.P.H.
Cathy L. Miller, R.N., Ph.D.

5 Emergency Department Management of
Trafficked Persons 65
Zheng Ben Ma, M.D.
Hanni Stoklosa, M.D., M.P.H.

6 Managing Trafficked Persons With
Comorbid Medical Conditions. 79
Rachel Robitz, M.D.
Amy Gajaria, M.D., FRCPC

7 General Principles of Care for
Trafficked Persons 91
Kimberly S.G. Chang, M.D., M.P.H.
Robert P. Marlin, M.D., Ph.D., M.P.H.

8 Responding to Trafficked Persons in
Health Care Settings: PATIENT-CENTERED,
SURVIVOR-CENTERED CARE 119
Susie B. Baldwin. M.D., M.P.H., FACPM
Holly Austin Gibbs, B.A.
Jordan Greenbaum, M.D.
Cathy L. Miller, R.N., Ph.D.

9 Care Management of Trafficked Persons
With Substance Use Disorders 133
Yasmine Omar, Ph.D.
Gabriela Austgen, M.D.
Nidal Moukaddam, M.D., Ph.D.

10 General and Specific Psychotherapy
Considerations for Managing Trafficked
Adults 149
Temilola Salami, Ph.D.
Grace Boland, B.A.
Christina Engelken, M.A.

11 Child Sex and Labor Trafficking 169
Jordan Greenbaum, M.D.

12 Cultural Aspects in the Assessment and
Management of Trafficked Persons 193
Ido Lurie, M.D., M.P.H.
Elana Cohn, M.D.
Ortal Slobodin, Ph.D.

13 The Clinician as Advocate: CONFIDENTIALITY
AND REPORTING REQUIREMENTS 213
Shea M. Rhodes, J.D.
Stephanie Mersch

14 Survivor Voices: CASE SCENARIOS OF LABOR
AND SEX TRAFFICKING 225
Holly Austin Gibbs, B.A.
Makini Chisolm-Straker, M.D., M.P.H.

Index 253

About the Editors

John Coverdale, M.B. Ch.B., M.D., M.Ed., FRANZCP, is professor of psychiatry and medical ethics at Baylor College of Medicine in Houston, Texas; serves as deputy editor of *Academic Psychiatry* and associate editor of *Academic Medicine*; and co-directs the anti-human trafficking program at Baylor College of Medicine. He has published more than 250 manuscripts in peer-reviewed journals on topics especially related to the care of vulnerable populations, professionalism, and medical education. He has won many awards, including the Vestermark Award for excellence, creativity, and leadership in psychiatric education (2016) and the Association of American Medical Colleges Presidential Award, the Alpha Omega Alpha Robert J. Glaser Distinguished Teacher Award (2017).

Mollie R. Gordon, M.D., is an associate professor in the Menninger Department of Psychiatry and Behavioral Sciences at Baylor College of Medicine in Houston, Texas, where she is a co-director of the Anti-Human Trafficking Program. She is a co-chair of the American Medical Women's Association Physicians Against the Trafficking of Humans, is on the HEAL trafficking speakers bureau, and has opined for the Office of Trafficking in Persons. Recently, she founded BCM Division of Global Mental Health to treat survivors of torture, trafficking, and mass violence atrocities. She has published numerous peer-reviewed articles and won numerous awards for her work.

Phuong T. Nguyen, Ph.D., is an associate professor in the Menninger Department of Psychiatry and Behavioral Sciences at Baylor College of Medicine. He is director of psychology services at Ben Taub Hospital and the program director of the BCM Anti-Human Trafficking Program. Additionally, he serves as the training director for the BCM Psychology Internship Program and the Ben Taub Hospital/BCM Psychology Postdoctoral Fellowship Program, which includes the country's first formal psychology postdoctoral fellowship track specializing in anti-human trafficking work. At BCM, Dr. Nguyen enjoys a mixture of leadership, training, clinical, and research activities. Given his refugee background, his clinical and research interests stem from his desire to better understand and address psychological difficulties experienced by historically underserved and marginalized groups, especially racial and ethnic minorities, refugees, internally displaced and homeless individuals, and human trafficking survivors.

DISCLOSURE OF COMPETING INTERESTS

The volume editors have indicated that they have no financial interests or other affiliations that represent or could appear to represent a competing interest with the contributions to this book.

Contributors

Gabriela Austgen, M.D.
PGY-3, Baylor College of Medicine, Houston, Texas

Susie B. Baldwin, M.D., M.P.H., FACPM
Medical Director, Office of Women's Health, Los Angeles County Department of Public Health, Los Angeles, California; President, HEAL Trafficking

Grace Boland, B.A.
Clinical Psychology Doctoral Student, Department of Psychology, Sam Houston State University, Huntsville, Texas

Ronald Chambers, M.D., FAAFP
Program Director, Dignity Health Family Medicine Residency Program, Methodist Hospital of Sacramento, Sacramento, California

Kimberly S.G. Chang, M.D., M.P.H.
Family Physician, Human Trafficking and Healthcare Policy Fellow, Asian Health Services, Oakland, California

Makini Chisolm-Straker, M.D., M.P.H.
Assistant Professor of Emergency Medicine, Icahn School of Medicine at Mount Sinai, New York; Co-founder, HEAL Trafficking, New York, New York

Elana Cohn, M.D.
Resident Physician, Institute of Family Health and Family Medicine, Mount Sinai Hospital, New York, New York

Christina Engelken, M.A.
Applied Psychology Graduate Student, Department of Psychology, Southern Illinois University, Carbondale, Illinois

Amy Gajaria, M.D., FRCPC
Assistant Professor, Department of Psychiatry, University of Toronto; Staff Psychiatrist, Child, Youth, and Emerging Adult Program, Centre for Addiction and Mental Health, Toronto, Ontario, Canada

Holly Austin Gibbs, B.A.
Patient Care Services Program Director, Violence and Human Trafficking Prevention and Response Program, CommonSpirit Health, Las Vegas, Nevada; Advisory Council Member, HEAL Trafficking

Jordan Greenbaum, M.D.
Medical Director, Global Initiative for Child Health & Well-Being, International Centre for Missing & Exploited Children; Medical Director, Institute on Healthcare and Human Trafficking, Stephanie V. Blank Center for Safe and Healthy Children, Children's Healthcare of Atlanta, Atlanta, Georgia; HEAL Trafficking

Ido Lurie, M.D., M.P.H.
Adult Outpatient Clinic Director, Shalvata Mental Health Center, Hod Hasharon, Israel; Clinical Senior Lecturer, Department of Psychiatry, Sackler School of Medicine, Tel Aviv University, Tel Aviv, Israel

Zheng Ben Ma, M.D.
Emergency Department Administrative Fellow, Partners Healthcare/Harvard Medical School; Emergency Physician, Department of Emergency Medicine, Brigham and Women's Hospital, Boston, Massachusetts

Robert P. Marlin, M.D., Ph.D., M.P.H.
Chief, Metta Health Center, Lowell Community Health Center, Lowell, Massachusetts

Stephanie Mersch
J.D. Candidate, Charles Widger School of Law, Villanova University, Villanova, Pennsylvania

Cathy L. Miller, R.N., Ph.D.
Associate Professor, University of Texas at Tyler; Co-Chair, Texas Coastal Bend Border Region Human Trafficking Task Force; Director of Research and Scholarship—United Nations Global Strategic Operatives for the Eradication of Human Trafficking, New Yor, New York; Member, Research Committee, HEAL Trafficking

Nidal Moukaddam, M.D., Ph.D.
Associate Professor, Baylor College of Medicine, Houston, Texas

Yasmine Omar, Ph.D.
Assistant Professor, Baylor College of Medicine, Houston, Texas

Frances Recknor, L.C.S.W., Dr.P.H.
Clinical Assistant Professor, Menninger Department of Psychiatry and Behavioral Sciences, Baylor College of Medicine, Houston, Texas

Shea M. Rhodes, J.D.
Director and Co-Founder, Villanova Law Institute to Address Commercial Sexual Exploitation

Rachel Robitz, M.D.
Health Sciences Assistant Clinical Professor, Department of Psychiatry and Behavioral Sciences, University of California Davis, Sacramento, California

Temilola Salami, Ph.D.
Assistant Professor of Clinical Psychology, Department of Psychology, Sam Houston State University, Huntsville, Texas

Ortal Slobodin, Ph.D.
Senior Lecturer, Department of Education, Ben-Gurion University, Beer-Sheva, Israel

Hanni Stoklosa, M.D., M.P.H.
Director, Global Women's Health Fellowship, Mary Horrigan Connors Center for Women's Health and Gender Biology, Brigham and Women's Hospital/Harvard Medical School; Emergency Physician, Department of Emergency Medicine, Brigham and Women's Hospital; Executive Director, HEAL Trafficking, Boston, Massachusetts

Melissa I.M. Torres, Ph.D., M.S.W.
Research Faculty, Assistant Professor, Menninger Department of Psychiatry and Behavioral Services, Baylor College of Medicine, Houston, Texas

DISCLOSURE OF COMPETING INTERESTS

The following contributors have indicated that they have no financial interests or other affiliations that represent or could appear to represent a competing interest with the contributions to this book:

Kimberly S. G. Chang, M.D., M.P.H.
Makini Chisolm-Straker, M.D., M.P.H.
Amy Gajaria, M.D., FRCPC
Holly Austin Gibbs, B.A.
Jordan Greenbaum, M.D.
Ido Lurie, M.D., M.P.H.
Zheng Ben Ma, M.D.
Robert P. Marlin, M.D., Ph.D., M.P.H.
Cathy L. Miller, R.N., Ph.D.
Frances Recknor, L.C.S.W., Dr.P.H.
Rachel Robitz, M.D.
Hanni Stoklosa, M.D., M.P.H.

Preface

This is the first book focused exclusively on human trafficking and mental health. The number of people, male and female, who are sex or labor trafficked, whom we see in our psychiatry service astounds us. At the time of this writing, we have formally identified, in the past year alone, close to 100 trafficked persons in our small 20-bed inpatient psychiatry unit, and the rate of those identified seems to be climbing. We have therefore been building our resources and interventional programs and applying for funding to support these programs. In addition, we have been engaging in research and scholarly writing. This book is an offshoot of our efforts to meaningfully address the problem of human trafficking.

Our book is inspired by our patients. We truly admire them for their courage and resilience and for what they have taught us. We are outraged by the horrific crime and human rights violation of human trafficking. Every case is tragic, and we are driven to help those harmed and to do something more to counter human trafficking.

We are also inspired by our wonderful colleagues who have contributed so much to this book. Our authors are all experts on human trafficking, and their contributions are outstanding. Without their commitment to the pursuit of excellence in their work, this book would not be the robust resource that it is.

We intend this book to be an educational and clinical resource for mental health practitioners as well as clinicians from any discipline who might encounter trafficked persons (which, essentially, is all of us in the health care field). We also intend it to be an educational resource. Thus, each chapter begins with a clinical case example and an inspirational quote to contextualize the material. In each chapter, goals are set forth, content is summarized, and take-away pearls and pointers are presented. Tables and figures serve as visual aids to the understanding and retention of the material.

There are 14 chapters. The first four address epidemiology and screening. In Chapter 1, "Becoming a Trafficked Person," Ronald

Chambers presents epidemiological data and an overview of the factors that contribute to becoming trafficked and some of the associated consequences and explores our role as health professionals in combating trafficking. In Chapter 2, "Epidemiology of Human Trafficking," Melissa Torres presents additional epidemiological data with a special emphasis on the importance of starting with clear definitions. In Chapter 3, "By the Right Name," Makini Chisolm-Straker provides an academic discussion of the processes of screening, including the importance of understanding the concepts of sensitivity and specificity. In Chapter 4, "Barriers to Identification of Trafficked Persons in Health Care Settings," Frances Recknor, Hanni Stoklosa, and Cathy Miller inform us about potential barriers to the identification of trafficked persons in relation to our organizational systems, to providers, and to the individuals themselves, given that an understanding of these obstacles is necessary when developing effective screening programs.

The second group of four chapters discusses general and specific management principles in different settings. In Chapter 5, "Emergency Department Management of Trafficked Persons," Zheng Ben Ma and Hanni Stoklosa stress the importance of a sensitive, trauma-informed, and integrated care approach to emergency room management, while emphasizing the priority to attend to medical needs first. In Chapter 6, "Managing Trafficked Persons With Comorbid Medical Conditions," Rachel Robitz and Amy Gajaria focus on the clinician management of adults and children with comorbid conditions. In Chapter 7, "General Principles of Care for Trafficked Persons," Kimberly Chang and Robert Marlin emphasize the importance of integrating primary care and behavioral health programs. This includes addressing substance use, providing trauma-informed care and safety planning, and managing chronic diseases, reproductive health, and concomitant substance use disorders, among other topics. In Chapter 8, "Responding to Human Trafficking in Health Care Settings," Susie Baldwin, Holly Gibbs, Jordan Greenbaum, and Cathy Miller describe in more detail the principles of a trauma-informed approach under the headings of privacy, education, asking, respecting, and responding.

The next four chapters focus on more specific topics such as managing persons with substance use disorders, issues pertaining to children, psychotherapeutic principles, and cultural issues. In Chapter 9, "Care Management of Trafficked Persons With Substance Use Disorders," Yasmine Omar, Gabriela Austgen, and Nidal Moukaddam discuss relevant diagnostic and treatment considerations. These include the importance of identifying and addressing countertransference feelings that may influence treatment. In Chapter 10, "General and Specific Psychotherapy Considerations for Managing Trafficked Adults," Temilola Salami, Grace Boland, and Christina Engelken discuss psychotherapeutic considerations pertinent to trafficked persons. This is an important topic about which little has been previously written. In Chapter 11, "Child Sex and Labor Trafficking," Jordan Greenbaum presents a comprehensive discussion of child sex and labor trafficking. In Chapter 12, "Cultural Aspects in the Assessment and Management of Trafficked Persons," Ido Lurie, Elana Cohn, and Ortal Slobodin describe some of the very complex cultural factors that are critical in the diagnosis and treatment of trafficked persons.

The final two chapters address topics such as advocacy, confidentiality, and reporting requirements. In Chapter 13, "The Clinician as Advocate," Shea Rhodes and Stephanie Mersch describe our role as advocates for trafficked persons, particularly as it relates to legal and ethical reporting requirements for adult and child patients. In Chapter 14, "Survivor Voices," Holly Gibbs and Makini Chisolm-Straker present 10 informative and true cases of how trafficked persons experienced and reacted to health care settings. The authors provide useful questions as prompts to promote our learning about how to identify and optimally care for these persons. For example, they ask, What more would clinicians find if they only took the time and looked beneath the surface?

It was a tremendous honor, as well as a solemn responsibility, to edit this book. We are indebted to the trafficked persons who have taught us so much. Every one of their stories is heartbreaking. We are also indebted to our colleagues who have authored these wonderful chapters and to their commitment to end the scourge of human trafficking. We hope that their work will assist you, dear readers, in your own work with trafficked persons.

With our sincerest thanks,

John H. Coverdale, M.B. Ch.B., M.D., M.Ed., FRANZCP
Mollie R. Gordon, M.D.
Phuong T. Nguyen, Ph.D.

CHAPTER 1

Becoming a Trafficked Person

Ronald Chambers, M.D., FAAFP

> ...for the first time in a long time I have hope for a future.
> —*Survivor, Dignity Health Medical Safe Haven clinic*

WHO ARE THE VICTIMS OF HUMAN TRAFFICKING?

The trafficking of humans, also called modern slavery, is an egregious violation of human rights and is one of the fastest growing crimes in the world, affecting more than 40 million people globally today (International Labour Organization 2017). The United Nations defines "trafficking in persons," or human trafficking, as

> the recruitment, transportation, transfer, harbouring or receipt of persons, by means of the threat or use of force or other forms of coercion, of abduction, of fraud, of deception, of the abuse of power or of a position of vulnerability or of the giving or receiving of payments or benefits to achieve the consent of a person having control over another person, for the purpose of exploitation. (United Nations Office on Drugs and Crime 2018)

Under this broad definition, human trafficking encompasses multiple illicit acts, including sex trafficking, forced labor, debt bondage, and other forms of involuntary servitude. In response to the growing threat and incidence of human trafficking, the United States passed the federal Trafficking Victims Protection Act of 2000 (TVPA; P.L. 106-386), which established tools and guidelines for the protection of victims, prosecution of perpetrators, and prevention of trafficking acts in the United States. Despite these protections, the U.S. Department of State estimates that 14,500–17,500 people are trafficked into the

United States each year (U.S. Department of State 2004). In addition, up to half of the trafficked persons population in the United States may be made up of U.S. citizens (National Human Trafficking Hotline 2018). Trafficked persons have been identified in every U.S. state and are especially prevalent in California, Texas, and New York (Lillie 2013). The Global Slavery Index estimates that as of 2016, there were approximately 403,000 people living in modern slavery within the United States, a prevalence of about 1.3 trafficked persons per thousand U.S. residents (Walk Free Foundation 2018).

Modern slavery occurs in every region of the world; however, it is most prevalent in Africa and East Asia (International Labour Organization 2017), with several countries listed as tier 3 (governments that do not meet TVPA standards and are making no effort to do so), including Russia, Iran, China, and North Korea (U.S. Department of State 2018). Because of strong anti-trafficking policies and the vigilant stance of the U.S. justice system, the United States is considered a tier 1 country in full compliance with the TVPA, and along with many western European countries, Canada, and Australia, it ranks among the most resolute of countries attempting to combat human trafficking, with one of the highest trafficker prosecution rates worldwide (U.S. Department of State 2018). Despite advances in minimizing human trafficking by punishing its perpetrators, there is a great need worldwide to better understand and support the survivors of human trafficking, especially within the health care system.

To begin to combat human trafficking, we must first understand who trafficked persons are. Importantly, there is no single profile of a trafficked person. In the United States, they include men, women, and children from all backgrounds and nationalities (National Human Trafficking Hotline 2018). Human trafficking is often conflated with human smuggling (U.S. Department of Justice 2018); however, whereas smuggling involves the unlawful transportation of a person, trafficking does not necessarily involve human transportation—only the forced exploitation of a person for sexual acts or labor. In the United States, trafficked persons have been identified in rural, suburban, and urban areas of all 50 states and include both minors and adults (National Human Trafficking Hotline 2018; National Human Trafficking Resource Center 2019a). Trafficked persons can come from all socioeconomic backgrounds, education levels, and demographic settings. They include documented and undocumented persons, migrants, and refugees. Some trafficked persons continue to interact in their communities and society, while others are hidden and imprisoned out of view (National Human Trafficking Hotline 2018).

This diversity of backgrounds and experiences makes human trafficking difficult to identify and therefore difficult to fight. However, although trafficked persons can be just about anyone, there are certain risk factors that increase vulnerability to trafficking.

PUSH AND PULL: RISK FACTORS FOR HUMAN TRAFFICKING

With increased study and understanding of victims and their traffickers, several contributing risk factors, circumstances, and vulnerabilities that lead to a higher susceptibility for human trafficking have been identified. Both "push" and "pull" factors exist: some risk factors push people into trafficking situations, whereas others pull them in (Figure 1–1).

Push Factors: Background and Experience

Many of the push factors relate to one's background, history, and experiences—some of which may harken back to early childhood. Some of the most common self-reported risk factors for human trafficking include poverty and economic insecurity, homelessness, runaway status, substance abuse, and prior childhood abuse and neglect (Polaris 2019a). In youth and minor trafficking, homelessness and runaway or "throw-away" status is a strong risk factor for being trafficked, with some studies estimating that more than half to, in some cases, more than 90% of sex trafficked minors are runaways (Choi 2015; National Human Trafficking Hotline 2019b; U.S. Department of Health and Human Services 2009). Other risk factors include factors that can lead to a sense of isolation or not fitting in. These can include LGBTQIA (lesbian, gay, bisexual, transgender, queer/questioning, intersex, asexual) status, lack of family or other social support structures, depression and mental illness, learning and developmental disabilities, and physical disabilities (Lo and Chambers 2016). Many trafficked persons suffer from previous physical, verbal, emotional, or sexual abuse and may experience psychological repercussions from these prior experiences as well (National Human Trafficking Hotline 2019a; UNICEF USA 2017). Undocumented migrants, refugees, and other foreign nationals who do not speak the native language are also at increased risk for trafficking (Weller 2014). Commonly, a multitude of factors are at play to push people into the life of trafficking, making individuals who are experiencing several of these factors simultaneously potentially the most vulnerable population for victimhood.

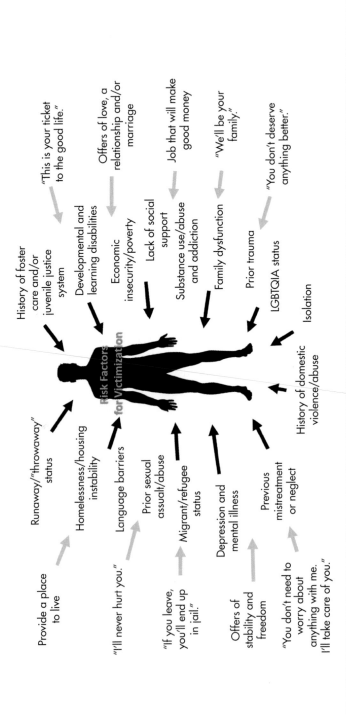

FIGURE 1–1. Common "push and pull" risk factors for human trafficking victimization.

Push factors (*black arrows*) often originate in the victim's background and experiences, including socioeconomic status, family situation, and previous trauma and abuse. Pull factors (*shaded arrows*) are often perpetuated by traffickers and used to coerce victims into trafficking situations. LGTBQIA=Lesbian, gay, transgender, bisexual, queer/questioning, intersex, asexual.

Pull Factors: Coercion Techniques of Traffickers

Traffickers also employ a variety of tactics to coerce and induce their victims into trafficking situations. To understand many of the "pull" factors that draw people into trafficking situations, we must understand the coercive tactics that traffickers use. These techniques are often tailored to the victim. Traffickers get to know and are sometimes deeply involved with their victims, often posing as romantic partners or supportive friends, and use psychological manipulation and feigned affection to induce them into the life (see Figure 1–1) (Baldwin et al. 2015; Polaris 2019b; Withers 2016). They may also make promises to their victims of economic security, a good job and steady income, or a home. Perpetrators may make trafficked persons economically dependent on them and may threaten their victims with the loss of that support or stability if they do not comply with their demands or if they attempt to leave (Polaris 2019b). In cases of undocumented migrants or refugees, the trafficker may threaten the victim with notifying the authorities, which could result in jail time and/or deportation. Trafficked persons often report fear of the authorities and legal repercussions as a reason for not leaving their traffickers (National Human Trafficking Resource Center 2013, 2019a; United Nations Office on Drugs and Crime 2016). Traffickers may also use addictive substances to entice their victims to comply with their demands and often combine positive and negative reinforcement as a means of control (National Institute on Drug Abuse for Teens 2017; Office for Victims of Crime, Training and Technical Assistance Center 2019; Stoklosa et al. 2017). In many cases, traffickers use multiple coercive techniques to maintain control of their victims (Baldwin et al. 2015).

One of the most difficult consequences of traffickers' abuse is the experience of trauma bonding. *Trauma bonding* is a psychological phenomenon whereby victims form an unhealthy emotional attachment to their abusers. It is observed in many situations, including domestic violence, child abuse, hostage situations, and human trafficking (National Domestic Violence Hotline 2019; Raghavan and Doychak 2015; Reid et al. 2013). Trauma bonding has been explained as a product of interpersonal trauma during which the perpetrator provokes fear in the trafficked person that in turn elicits feelings of gratitude for being allowed to survive or for any perceived kindness or affection given by the abuser. Trauma bonding is not well understood, and there is currently no widely accepted theory to explain how perpetrators emotionally bind their victims to them, making it a complicated issue for trafficked persons and their caregivers to overcome (National Domestic Violence Hotline 2019). People experiencing trauma bonding may be compelled to protect or defend their captor or even return to them after leaving (National Domestic Violence Hotline 2019; Raghavan and Doychak 2015; Reid et al. 2013). Trauma bonding represents a challenging and critical hurdle both for health care providers and community support groups that are attempting to protect and treat trafficking survivors and for law enforcement officials who are striving to protect survivors and to prosecute offenders.

WHY IS HUMAN TRAFFICKING CONSIDERED A PUBLIC HEALTH ISSUE?

Human trafficking is increasingly being recognized as a public health issue by public officials, community organizations, and professional health care associations. The American Academy of Family Physicians officially recognizes the enormous health impacts of human trafficking and encourages cooperation between health care providers, community organizations, and law enforcement to identify, protect, and prevent victimization and to provide trauma-informed care for survivors (American Academy of Family Physicians 2019). Additionally, the American Psychological Association passed a resolution in 2017 on human trafficking in the United States that encourages funding for research on human trafficking, especially of women and girls, to better understand the risk factors for human trafficking, the psychological impact of trafficking on trafficked individuals, and the impact of societal biases on survivors. The resolution also supports evidence-based training of health care professionals in trauma-informed care (American Psychological Association 2017). The American Medical Association, American Hospital Association, American Medical Women's Association, and American Public Health Association, along with other local, state, and national associations and societies, similarly support additional resources for the study and awareness of human trafficking as a public health concern (American Hospital Association 2019; American Medical Association 2015; American Medical Women's Association 2019; American Public Health Association 2015).

The usefulness of the term *public health crisis* is debated by many experts in the field, given the implications and concern about a dramatic yet short-sighted societal response. However, at a survivor-centered level, the term *crisis* is certainly appropriate for an individual or a community.

Physical and Psychological Consequences of Human Trafficking

Human trafficking can have long-term, lasting health consequences for survivors, including physical and psychological impacts. Trafficked persons may not have access to routine, preventive medical care, including immunizations, physical exams, and dental care. Trafficked individuals frequently present with injuries, sexually transmitted infections and diseases, signs of physical trauma such as bruising and scarring, malnutrition, untreated fractures, and signs of substance abuse such as track marks and abnormal or impaired cognition and behavior (National Human Trafficking Resource Center 2019a). Many of these signs may be seen by law enforcement officials and health care providers as "red flag" evidence of human trafficking and abuse. Additional long-term physical ailments can include chronic pain, cardiovascular and respiratory diseases, neurological disorders, and a variety of diseases associated with prolonged malnutrition, fatigue, and overwork (Lederer and Wetzel 2014; National Human Trafficking Resource Center 2019a).

Survivors also overwhelmingly experience psychological trauma during their trafficking, which can lead to several long-term mental health consequences (Ottisova et al. 2016). A recent study of sex trafficking reported that 98% of the more than 100 survivors interviewed had experienced at least one psychological disorder during captivity (Lederer and Wetzel 2014). Survivors commonly report psychological issues, including anxiety, depression, disordered eating, chronic fatigue, insomnia, nightmares, flashbacks, low self-esteem, acute stress, personality disorders, and acute, chronic, or complex PTSD (Altun et al. 2017; Lederer and Wetzel 2014; Ottisova et al. 2016). Sadly, suicide attempts and other forms of self-harm are not uncommon among survivors of trafficking (Altun et al. 2017; Lederer and Wetzel 2014). As with the risk factors noted above, many trafficked persons experience multiple physical and psychological consequences trafficking long after they have escaped their abusers.

Given the trauma and abuse that survivors of human trafficking suffer, one of the consequences of trafficking that may be hardest to understand is *recidivism*—returning to trafficking situations. Despite the efforts of support groups, organizations, and health care providers, survivors do occasionally backslide into their former way of life, and a number of factors are involved, many of them the same ones that pushed or pulled the person into trafficking situations in the first place (Fowler et al. 2010). Trauma bonding may play a significant role in pulling survivors back to their captors, especially if those captors still offer psychological incentives such as affection, stability, love, or support, as well promises of fulfilling practical needs such as income and housing. As survivors of all kinds of trauma report, the road to recovery is challenging, and recovery from human trafficking is no different. To care for these individuals and reduce recidivism rates, a greater understanding of trafficked persons' psychological triggers and drivers is needed.

Persistence of Human Trafficking

Unfortunately, despite efforts to better understand and develop techniques to prevent this crime, human trafficking is the second largest criminal industry in the world after the drug trade and is considered by officials to be the fastest growing. There are several factors that make fighting human trafficking difficult and allow it to persist throughout the world today. First, trafficking is often a hidden crime, occurring in the midst of our communities without our knowledge. For the many reasons described above, trafficked persons are often unwilling or unable to report their traffickers or seek help from authorities (National Human Trafficking Resource Center 2019c; Tyldum 2010). Indeed, we may not know the true extent or incidence of human trafficking because trafficked persons rarely elect to self-report or may not even self-identify (National Human Trafficking Resource Center 2019a). Second, human trafficking is a lucrative trade garnering an estimated $150 billion in illegal profits annually (International Labour Organization 2014). There is great financial incentive for perpetrators to enter and remain in the trafficking industry, and high profits come with relatively low risks (Institute for Faith, Work, and Economics 2016; International Labour Organization 2014; National Human Trafficking Hotline 2018). Finally, the myths, misconceptions, and misunderstandings surrounding human trafficking and its victims may be the largest contributors to the persistence of human trafficking (Table 1–1). These misconceptions pose a challenge to public awareness and education about the risk factors and consequences of human trafficking and hinder enlistment of multiple participants in combating human trafficking and protecting trafficked persons.

TABLE 1–1.   Myths and misconceptions about human
trafficking and its victims

MYTH	FACT
Human trafficking does not occur in the United States or other developed countries.	Human trafficking occurs in all countries, including the United States.
Human trafficking victims are always undocumented or other foreign nationals.	Victims can be foreign nationals or U.S. citizens and may or may not be documented.
Human trafficking only happens in cities.	Trafficking occurs in urban, rural, and suburban areas.
Only women and children are victims of human trafficking.	Victims of human trafficking include both men and women and minors and adults.
Victims could just leave the trafficking situation whenever they want.	There are many factors that drive and keep victims in trafficking situations, including coercion, psychological manipulation, lack of resources, trauma bonding, and fear.
Trafficking does not have any long-term consequences for its victims.	Trafficking has several long-term physical and psychological impacts on victims, including sexually transmitted infections and diseases, chronic pain, depression, isolation, and PTSD.
Only homeless people and drug addicts are trafficked.	Homelessness and substance use/addiction are risk factors for victimization but do not characterize all potential victims.
There is nothing health care providers can do to prevent human trafficking or protect victims.	Health care providers can be a first line of defense to prevent trafficking and provide care that helps victims to heal and rehabilitate.

ROLE OF THE HEALTH CARE PROVIDER IN COMBATING HUMAN TRAFFICKING

With the increasing recognition and appreciation of the growing and lasting impacts of human trafficking, a call to action has arisen for health care providers to assist in combating human trafficking by identifying and providing trauma-informed and survivor-centered care to trafficked persons while giving them the resources to escape the bonds of trafficking and support their healing and rehabilitation. Human trafficking survivors are frequently seen by health care providers, but many go unrecognized, and therefore their special health and social needs are unaddressed (Lederer and Wetzel 2014; Lo and Chambers 2016). Earlier estimates suggest that anywhere from 30% to more than 80% of trafficked persons had contacted a health care provider while they were in captivity (Coalition to Abolish Slavery and Trafficking 2017; Lederer and Wetzel 2014; O'Callaghan 2012). Unfortunately, in one study, a staggering 97% of trafficked persons who had seen a health care professional reported that they did not receive any resources or information about trafficking and were never identified as survivors of trafficking (Coalition to Abolish Slavery and Trafficking 2017). This is troubling because survivors of trafficking have a multitude of specific physical and mental health care needs, as described earlier (see subsection "Physical and Psychological Consequences of Human Trafficking"). Because of the growing needs of this population, experts have called on the health care community to help address this public health concern (Zimmerman and Kiss 2017).

Health care professionals have the opportunity to provide a first line of defense in the prevention of trafficking (Greenbaum et al. 2018) and an ethical obligation to provide trauma-informed and culturally sensitive care to survivors (Rollins et al. 2017). Employment of a harm reduction model, similar to what has been used successfully for substance users and addicts (Harm Reduction Coalition 2019; Ritter and Cameron 2006), has shown promise for sex workers and victims of sex trafficking (Hickle and Hallett 2016; Rekart 2005). Not all individuals are ready or want to leave their trafficking situations, but they are deserving of equitable and respectful health care regardless. It is also important to remember that for many trafficked persons, health care providers offer the only opportunity to access the resources needed to help them out of the trafficking situation when they are ready. Health care providers are able and encouraged to pair with local community organizations, support groups, and trauma therapy providers who can ease the path to healing and rehabilitation. Providers may also have access to other survivors who can provide the expertise and guidance needed to provide better trauma-informed care to survivors and improve the success rate of survivor care and recovery.

The largest challenge facing the health care of trafficked persons is that providers often lack the training and education to care for this patient population. In one study of emergency department personnel, only 13% of study participants felt confident they could identify a trafficked individual, and fewer than 3% had ever received training in victim recognition (Chisolm-Straker and Richardson 2007). Barriers to health care providers' ability to identify and treat survivors of trafficking include lack of knowledge and awareness of human trafficking, misconceptions and cultural assumptions about trafficked persons, and a failure to apply trauma-informed care (Barrows and Finger 2008; Haynes 2004; Substance Abuse and Mental Health Services Administration 2014; Viergever et al. 2015). Fortunately, for survivors today, several programs now exist to disseminate information to and training for health care providers about how to identify trafficked persons and how to apply trauma-informed care that is sensitive to the patient's past experiences and maximizes healing and recovery while minimizing the risk of retraumatization. Tools have been developed that can help providers identify the red flags of human trafficking, thereby enabling them to provide adequate care and resources to their patients. These tools and techniques are discussed further in the chapters that follow.

Additionally, because the survivors of human trafficking come from all walks of life and from all backgrounds and experiences, there are many special considerations to keep in mind when treating these patients. Care must be taken to address human trafficking victims with mental health disorders, victims who are minors, pregnant victims, victims with substance use history, victims with comorbid health conditions, victims in the emergency department, victims who are refugees, victims who are LGBTQIA individuals, and others. These cases will be covered in subsequent chapters of this book. Overall, to provide the most beneficial care to survivors of human trafficking, health care providers must first understand who human trafficking patients are and the factors and experiences that influence their situation, as well as the physical, psychological, and social barriers and traumas that continue to shape their journey to healing and recovery.

CONCLUSION

Human trafficking is a global public health *issue* of national scale and a *crisis* at the patient-centered individual or community level. As human trafficking continues to expand, so too must the response of health care professionals who see and care for trafficked persons every day within the United States and worldwide. Although we have many times referred to these patients as "trafficked persons" or "survivors" throughout this chapter to avoid the stigmatization that is often associated with the term "victim" (similar to the usage of "persons experiencing homelessness" rather than "the homeless"), it is important to acknowledge that human trafficking is not and should never be normalized and to recognize that individuals who have experienced trafficking are in fact victims of an egregious crime perpetrated by their traffickers, even if they do not self-identify as and wish to avoid the term victim. It is important to speak to survivors of trafficking in terms that they are most comfortable with, following the harm reduction model, and to avoid victim blaming and stigmatization in order to help patients heal from their trauma. Conversely, the use of terms such as victim may promote growing societal awareness and empathy among the uninformed public (e.g., someone may have a preconception of an individual as "just a prostitute" that is dramatically altered if there is a realization that he or she may in fact be a victim of sex trafficking). Trafficking survivors come from all backgrounds and have often experienced multiple push and pull factors that have influenced their path through trafficking. Recognizing victims and survivors of human trafficking within the clinic and the unique physical and psychological needs of survivors and the role of health care professionals in providing victim-centered survivor and trauma-informed comprehensive care are crucial first steps in the battle against human trafficking and along the path to healing.

Pearls and Pointers

- Trauma-coerced attachment (trauma bonding) and its impact on the recovery of your patient should not be underestimated.
- Vicarious trauma is real. Techniques should be developed that mitigate it early in the treatment process.
- Clinicians should work with, learn from, and take the advice of survivors. Survivor-informed practices are key, and survivors should be paid for their expertise.

- Community agency collaboration will "make" the work we do with persons who have experienced exploitation. A lack of collaboration and multidisciplinary approaches will break it.
- Empathy, a term much overused in medicine, is necessary.

REFERENCES

American Academy of Family Physicians: Human trafficking. 2019. Available at: www.aafp.org/about/policies/all/human-trafficking.html. Accessed October 23, 2019.

American Hospital Association: Combating human trafficking. 2019. Available at: www.aha.org/combating-human-trafficking. Accessed October 23, 2019.

Altun S, Abas M, Zimmerman C, et al: Mental health and human trafficking: responding to survivors' needs. BJPsych Int 14(1):21–23, 2017 29093930

American Medical Association: Physicians response to victims of human trafficking H-65.966. 2015. Available at: https://policysearch.ama-assn.org/policyfinder/detail/H-65.966?uri=%2FAMADoc%2FHOD.xml-0-5095.xml. Accessed October 23, 2019.

American Medical Women's Association: Physicians Against the Trafficking of Humans (PATH). 2019. Available at: www.amwa-doc.org/our-work/initiatives/human-trafficking. Accessed October 23, 2019.

American Psychological Association: Resolution on human trafficking in the United States, especially of women and girls. February 2017. Available at: www.apa.org/about/policy/trafficking-women-girls. Accessed October 23, 2019.

American Public Health Association: Expanding and coordinating human trafficking-related public health research, evaluation, education, and prevention. November 3, 2015. Available at: www.apha.org/policies-and-advocacy/public-health-policy-statements/policy-database/2016/01/26/14/28/expanding-and-coordinating-human-trafficking-related-public-health-activities. Accessed October 23, 2019.

Baldwin SB, Fehrenbacher AE, Eisenman DP: Psychological coercion in human trafficking: an application of Biderman's framework. Qual Health Res 25(9):1171–1181, 2015 25371382

Barrows J, Finger R: Human trafficking and the healthcare professional. South Med J 101(5):521–524, 2008 18414161

Chisolm-Straker M, Richardson L: Assessment of emergency department (ED) provider knowledge about human trafficking victims in the ED. Academic Emergency Medicine 14(5 Suppl 1):S134, 2007

Choi KR: Risk factors for domestic minor sex trafficking in the United States: a literature review. J Forensic Nurs 11(2):66–76, 2015 25996431

Coalition to Abolish Slavery and Trafficking: Identification and referral for human trafficking survivors in health care settings: survey report. January 13, 2017. Available at: www.castla.org/wp-content/themes/castla/assets/files/Identification_and_Referral_in_Health_Care_Settings_survey_report_2017.pdf. Accessed October 23, 2019.

Fowler J, Che N, Fowler L: Innocence lost: the rights of human trafficking victims. Procedia: Social and Behavioral Sciences 2(2):1345–1349, 2010

Greenbaum VJ, Titchen K, Walker-Descartes I, et al: Multi-level prevention of human trafficking: the role of health care professionals. Prev Med 114:164–167, 2018 29981790

Harm Reduction Coalition: Principles of harm reduction. 2019. Available at: https://harmreduction.org/about-us/principles-of-harm-reduction. Accessed October 23, 2019.

Haynes DF: Used, abused, arrested and deported: extending immigration benefits to protect the victims of trafficking and to secure the prosecution of traffickers. Human Rights Quarterly 26(2):221–272, 2004

Hickle K, Hallett S: Mitigating harm: considering harm reduction principles in work with sexually exploited young people. Child Soc 30:302–313, 2016

Institute for Faith, Work, and Economics: The economics of human trafficking. April 12, 2016. Available at: https://tifwe.org/the-economics-of-human-trafficking. Accessed October 23, 2019.

International Labour Organization: Profits and poverty: the economics of forced labour. May 20, 2014. Available at: www.ilo.org/wcmsp5/groups/public/---ed_norm/---declaration/documents/publication/wcms_243391.pdf. Accessed October 23, 2019.

International Labour Organization: Global estimates of modern slavery: forced labour and forced marriage. September 19, 2017. Available at: www.ilo.org/wcmsp5/groups/public/---dgreports/---dcomm/documents/publication/wcms_575479.pdf. Accessed October 23, 2019.

Lederer LJ, Wetzel CA: The health consequences of sex trafficking and their implications for identifying victims in healthcare facilities. Annals of Health Law 23(1):61–87, 2014

Lillie M: Top 3 states for human trafficking (blog entry). Human Trafficking Search. 2013. Available at: https://humantraffickingsearch.org/top-3-states-for-human-trafficking. Accessed April 13, 2020.

Lo V, Chambers R: Human trafficking and the role of physicians. J Fam Med Community Health 3(3):1084, 2016

National Domestic Violence Hotline: Trauma bonds: what are they and how can we overcome them? 2019. Available at: www.thehotline.org/2018/07/31/trauma-bonds-what-are-they-and-how-can-we-overcome-them. Accessed October 23, 2019.

National Human Trafficking Hotline: Hotline statistics. December 31, 2018. Available at: https://humantraffickinghotline.org/states. Accessed October 23, 2019.

National Human Trafficking Hotline: Human trafficking. 2019a. Available at: https://humantraffickinghotline.org/type-trafficking/human-trafficking. Accessed October 23, 2019.

National Human Trafficking Hotline: The victims. 2019b. Available at: https://humantraffickinghotline.org/what-human-trafficking/human-trafficking/victims. Accessed October 23, 2019.

National Human Trafficking Resource Center: 2013 statistical overview. 2013. Available at: http://traffickingresourcecenter.org/sites/default/files/NHTRC%202013%20Statistical%20Overview.pdf. Accessed October 23, 2019.

National Human Trafficking Resource Center: Identifying victims of human trafficking fact sheet. 2019a. Available at: www.acf.hhs.gov/sites/default/files/orr/fact_sheet_identifying_victims_of_human_trafficking.pdf. Accessed October 23, 2019.

National Human Trafficking Resource Center: Identifying victims of human trafficking: what to look for in a healthcare setting. 2019b. Available at: https://humantraffickinghotline.org/sites/default/files/What%20to%20Look%20for%20during%20a%20Medical%20Exam%20-%20FINAL%20-%202-16-16_0.pdf. Accessed October 23, 2019.

National Human Trafficking Resource Center: The mindset of a human trafficking victim. 2019c. Available at: www.acf.hhs.gov/sites/default/files/orr/understanding_the_mindset_of_a_trafficking_victim_1.pdf. Accessed October 23, 2019.

National Institute on Drug Abuse for Teens: Human trafficking and drugs. June 19, 2017. Available at: https://teens.drugabuse.gov/blog/post/human-trafficking-and-drugs. Accessed October 23, 2019.

O'Callaghan MG: The health care professional as a modern abolitionist. Perm J 16(2):67–69, 2012 22745622

Office for Victims of Crime, Training and Technical Assistance Center: Human Trafficking Task Force e-Guide: substance abuse needs. 2019. Available at: www.ovcttac.gov/taskforceguide/eguide/4-supporting-victims/44-comprehensive-victim-services/mental-health-needs/substance-abuse-needs. Accessed October 23, 2019.

Ottisova L, Hemmings S, Howard LM, et al: Prevalence and risk of violence and the mental, physical and sexual health problems associated with human trafficking: an updated systematic review. Epidemiol Psychiatr Sci 25(4):317–341, 2016 27066701

Polaris: Sex trafficking in the U.S.: a closer look at U.S. citizen victims. 2019a. Available at: https://polarisproject.org/sites/default/files/us-citizen-sex-trafficking.pdf. Accessed October 23, 2019.

Polaris: The victims and traffickers. 2019b. Available at: https://polarisproject.org/victims-traffickers. Accessed October 23, 2019.

Raghavan C, Doychak K: Trauma-coerced bonding and victims of sex trafficking: where do we go from here? International Journal of Emergency Mental Health 17(2):583–587, 2015

Reid J, Haskell R, Dillahunt-Aspillaga C, et al: Trauma bonding and interpersonal violence. Faculty Publications, January 2013. Available at: https://digital.usfsp.edu/fac_publications/198. Accessed October 23, 2019.

Rekart ML: Sex-work harm reduction. Lancet 366(9503):2123–2134, 2005 16360791

Ritter A, Cameron J: A review of the efficacy and effectiveness of harm reduction strategies for alcohol, tobacco and illicit drugs. Drug Alcohol Rev 25(6):611–624, 2006 17132577

Rollins R, Gribble A, Barrett SE, et al: Who is in your waiting room? Health care professionals as culturally responsive and trauma-informed first responders to human trafficking. AMA J Ethics 19(1):63–71, 2017 28107157

Stoklosa H, MacGibbon M, Stoklosa J: Human trafficking, mental illness, and addiction: avoiding diagnostic overshadowing. AMA J Ethics 19(1):23–34, 2017 28107153

Substance Abuse and Mental Health Services Administration: SAMHSA's concept of trauma and guidance for a trauma-informed approach. July 2014. Available at: https://store.samhsa.gov/system/files/sma14-4884.pdf. Accessed October 23, 2019.

Trafficking Victims Protection Act of 2000, Pub. L. No. 106-386 (114 Stat. 1463–1491)

Tyldum G: Limitations in research on human trafficking. International Migration 48(5):1–13, 2010

UNICEF USA: Domestic violence and human trafficking. November 15, 2017. Available at: www.unicefusa.org/stories/domestic-violence-and-human-trafficking/33601. Accessed October 23, 2019.

United Nations Office on Drugs and Crime: Global report on trafficking in persons 2016. 2016. Available at: www.unodc.org/documents/data-and-analysis/glotip/2016_Global_Report_on_Trafficking_in_Persons.pdf. Accessed October 23, 2019.

United Nations Office on Drugs and Crime: Protocol to prevent, suppress, and punish trafficking in persons. July 26, 2018. Available at: www. unodc.org/unodc/en/human-trafficking/what-is-human-trafficking.html. Accessed October 23, 2019.

U.S. Department of Health and Human Services: Human trafficking into and within the United States: a review of the literature. Other populations at risk for trafficking: runaway and homeless youth. Office of the Assistant Secretary for Planning and Evaluation, August 30, 2009. Available at: https://aspe.hhs.gov/report/human-trafficking-and-within-united-states-review-literature/other-populations-risk-trafficking-runaway-and-homeless-youth. Accessed October 23, 2019.

U.S. Department of Justice: Human trafficking prosecution unit. October 18, 2018. Available at: www.justice.gov/crt/human-trafficking-prosecution-unit-htpu. Accessed October 23, 2019.

U.S. Department of State: Trafficking in persons report, June 2004. June 2004. Available at: www.state.gov/j/tip/rls/tiprpt/2004/34021.htm. Accessed October 23, 2019.

U.S. Department of State: Trafficking in persons report. June 2018. Available at: www.state.gov/wp-content/uploads/2019/01/282798.pdf. Accessed October 22, 2019.

Viergever RF, West H, Borland R, et al: Health care providers and human trafficking: what do they know, what do they need to know? Findings from the Middle East, the Caribbean, and Central America. Front Public Health 3(6):6, 2015 25688343

Walk Free Foundation: Global Slavery Index: United States. 2018. Available at: www.globalslaveryindex.org/2018/findings/country-studies/united-states/. Accessed October 23, 2019.

Weller S: Human trafficking and immigrant victims, in A Guide to Human Trafficking for State Courts. Edited by Martin JA. Human Trafficking and the State Courts Collaborative, July 2014. Available at: www.htcourts.org/wp-content/uploads/Ch-3_140725_NAC-M_Guide_OnlineVersion_v04.pdf. Accessed October 23, 2019.

Withers M: Psychological tactics used by human traffickers. Psychology Today, 2016. Available at: www.psychologytoday.com/us/blog/modern-day-slavery/201610/psychological-tactics-used-human-traffickers. Accessed October 23, 2019.

Zimmerman C, Kiss L: Human trafficking and exploitation: a global health concern. PLoS Med 14(11):e1002437, 2017 29166396

CHAPTER 2

Epidemiology of Human Trafficking

COMPLEXITIES AND INTERSECTIONS OF VULNERABILITY, RISK, AND EXPLOITATION

Melissa I. M. Torres, Ph.D., M.S.W.

> To affirm that men and women are persons and as persons should be free, and yet to do nothing tangible to make this affirmation a reality, is a farce.
>
> —*Paulo Freire* Pedagogy of the Oppressed *(1970)*

After a major hurricane, an immigrant day laborer sees that his work opportunities have increased drastically as clean up and rebuilding efforts begin in the region. His expertise is flooring, which is in high demand after the flooding, but he is also very experienced in remodeling and can perform many jobs for which there is a great need at the time. One day, he is approached by a contractor as he seeks work on the streets. A home is being remodeled, and the priority now is flooring. The day laborer has his own tools and, after discussing price, is selected by the contractor for the job. After the first day on the job, the contractor tells the day laborer that he does not have the full amount of cash for payment on that day but will pay him in installments as the project continues. The day laborer completes the job and charges the contractor, but the contractor doesn't pay him. While the contractor is arguing with the day laborer, he tells him to leave and refuses to let him back into the workplace, confiscating the day laborer's tools. When the day laborer tries to go back for his tools, the contractor calls the police and tells them that an undocumented man is trespassing, forcing the laborer to leave. The day laborer returns to his usual spot seeking work, knowing he might not get as much work now without his own tools and knowing that he may be maltreated or robbed of earnings again.

On December 10, 1948, the United Nations General Assembly proclaimed the Universal Declaration of Human Rights as the universal standard for fundamental human rights that all persons—regardless of nation, culture, or background—are afforded and that are to be universally protected (United Nations General Assembly 1948). The declaration comprises a preamble and 30 articles, with the first three articles addressing the universality of the declaration, equality, and liberty, respectively. Article 4 then addresses the first human rights violation of the declaration: "No one shall be held in slavery or servitude; slavery and the slave trade shall be prohibited in all their forms" (United Nations General Assembly 1948). Not being enslaved is, thus, a fundamental human right, making the enslavement of another person a human rights violation. The protection of human rights is essential to public health. Exploitation and the refusal of an individual's basic rights endanger both physical and mental health. Human trafficking is a human rights violation and should be considered a global health priority.

DEFINING HUMAN TRAFFICKING

Human trafficking has been termed "modern-day slavery" (Ngwe and Elechi 2012; Shadan 2006; Sigmon 2008). Separately from the aforementioned proclamation of slavery as a human rights violation, the United Nations defines human trafficking as

> the recruitment, transportation, transfer, harbouring or receipt of persons, by means of the threat or use of force or other forms of coercion, of abduction, of fraud, of deception, of the abuse of power or of a position of vulnerability or of the giving or receiving of payments or benefits to achieve the consent of a person having control over another person, for the purpose of exploitation. (United Nations General Assembly 2000)

The inclusion of various means of how the exploitation can occur in the definition is demonstrative of the intersecting and multidimensional nature of exploitation through force, fraud, and coercion.

The United States instituted its own similar policy of human trafficking the same year with the Trafficking Victims Protection Act of 2000, defining sex trafficking as "recruitment, harboring, transportation, provision, or obtaining of a person for the purpose of a commercial sex act"; "severe forms of trafficking in persons" for sex are defined as "sex trafficking in which the commercial sex act is induced by force, fraud, or coercion, or in which the person induced to perform such act has not attained 18 years of age." Severity of trafficking in persons for the purpose of labor is defined as "the recruitment, harboring, transportation, provision, or obtaining of a person for labor or services, through the use of force, fraud, or coercion for the purpose of subjection to involuntary servitude, peonage, debt bondage, or slavery" (P.L. 106-386). Regardless of this distinction between sex and labor, human trafficking is the exploitation of a person for the purpose of profiting from their compelled services of labor or commercial sex acts through the use of force, fraud, or coercion.

The approach to countering human trafficking, particularly in the United States, has long been to deem it a criminal act and a blight on society, rendering it something that needs to be addressed through both penal and charitable responses. These strategies are based on the overwhelming focus on sex trafficking and its conflation as the only or most notorious typology of human exploitation, although studies and surveys have shown that human trafficking for the purpose of labor exploitation is far more prevalent worldwide and occurs through more business models than sexual exploitation (Busch-Armendariz et al. 2016; International Labour Organization 2017; Polaris 2017; Weitzer 2014; Zhang 2012; Zimmerman and Kiss 2017).

It is also important to note that definitions are not globally uniform. For example, some individuals and governments regard commercial sexual services as a form of labor that, when exploited, constitutes a form of labor trafficking (Weitzer 2014; Zimmerman and Kiss 2017). Moreover, different forms of exploitation have different population distributions, each of these phenomena is likely to affect subgroups differently, and trafficking-related acts are very diverse (Kiss and Zimmerman 2019). A lack of uniform definitions can complicate an understanding of the factors that lead to exploitation and trafficking. It is also important to understand the various types of trauma experienced by victims and survivors.

On a global scale, the International Labour Organization estimates that 24.9 million people are trafficked, with 20.1 million exploited for labor or state-imposed forced labor and 4.8 million exploited for commercial sex in 2016 alone (International Labour Organization 2017). The Global Slavery Index puts the global estimate at 35 million, with forced labor being the largest typology (Walk Free Foundation 2018). Interestingly, this rate is similar to global HIV estimates from the World Health Organization, which put the number of persons living with HIV/AIDS at about 40 million (World Health Organization 2018). With these numbers, the World Health Organization defined HIV as a global epidemic and health crisis; similar numbers, prevalence, and emergency health needs are occurring among victims and survivors of human trafficking. Federal and regional reports in the United States have also estimated the number of human trafficking persons to range from tens of thousands to hundreds of thousands for both sex and labor trafficking (Busch-Armendariz et al. 2016; U.S. Department of State 2017). Because of the many limitations of the available data related to the methodologies of research and reporting processes, these estimates are usually considered to be conservative with respect to the actual incidence of exploitation for commercial sex or labor. With so many challenges in conducting research on human trafficking and surveys with victims and survivors, much of the data explores prevalence and incidence, with less attention given to population-based data.

Data are scarce concerning morbidity and comorbidities, including concomitant mental health disorders, and yet such data are crucial to better understanding the intersections of health (including mental health) with the trafficking experience. Some attention has been given to reproductive health and sexually transmitted illnesses as they relate to sex trafficking (Decker 2013; Falb et al. 2011). Less attention has been given to occupational health or the social determinants of health among those most at risk of exploitative work, such as those in poverty, low-wage workers, immigrants and migrants, and temporary/transient laborers. A global estimate of the economic impact of work-related injuries and illnesses (not counting fatalities) was calculated in U.S. dollars as $2.8 trillion in 2013 (International Labour Organization 2013). Estimates, however, have not been explored in terms of occupational injuries, illness, or fatalities related to labor exploitation and trafficking.

NUANCES OF HUMAN TRAFFICKING: EPIDEMIOLOGY AND CYCLES OF VIOLENCE

In 2015, the United Nations set 17 sustainable development goals as the basis for its 2030 Agenda for Sustainable Development. The focus on social and economic inequalities included poverty and climate; decent work as an important factor in sustainable development was also considered. Goal 8, for example, is to "promote sustained, inclusive and sustainable economic growth, full and productive employment and decent work for all" (United Nations General Assembly 2015). Most victims and survivors of labor or sex trafficking experience abuse, violence, hazardous working conditions, and risk long-term effects on their physical and mental health (Falb et al. 2011; Kiss et al. 2015). High-risk work environments are more prevalent in impoverished communities and developing countries and often occur when low-cost labor is sought (International Labour Organization 2013). Thus, the economic drivers of trafficking and the related vulnerabilities must be addressed through preventive efforts.

The business of human trafficking is burgeoning because it is financially rewarding for perpetrators. The basis of the exploitation depends on a relationship in which one individual has the opportunity and motive to profit from another's vulnerability. Human trafficking is a form of interpersonal violence that can be viewed as compounded acts of violence that intersect with systems of oppression (Lindhorst and Tajima 2008). The domestic violence and intimate partner violence fields have approached these forms of violence as preventable public health problems (Lindhorst and Tajima 2008); a gender-based report found that up to 69% of women worldwide reported being subjected to intimate partner violence at some point in their lifetime (World Health Organization et al. 2013). Behavioral factors have become a focus in violence research (Hachtel et al. 2018), including the behavioral factors associated with traffickers (Reid 2016; Troshynski and Blank 2007). Understanding these factors and viewing human trafficking as preventable are critical to preventive efforts.

RANGE OF EXPLOITATION

The media has tended to focus on the commercial sexual exploitation of children or has tended to portray labor trafficking as specifically an immigrant issue. A narrowly focused media can mislead the public about the extent of the problem. Similarly, a lack of clarity in the media about the phenomenon of human trafficking can also cause the public to fail to appreciate the extent of the problem, which in turn can limit efforts to mobilize and confront it.

Focusing on the determinants of health within communities experiencing violence can enable better detection, treatment, and prevention of human trafficking. Some violence prevention programs, including sex worker outreach programs, have adopted a harm reduction approach (Panchanadeswaran et al. 2008; Wood et al. 2019). Furthermore, identifying and detecting the many methods and degrees of exploitation will assist in the identification of victims.

The necessary elements that define the exploitation in human trafficking—force, fraud, coercion—are themselves indicative of the many ways and varying degrees to which someone can be exploited for profit. Further exploration and understanding of these elements, especially through the perspectives of victims and perpetrators, is needed in both research and clinical approaches. Trafficked persons do not always disclose their situation in health care settings (Leslie 2018), although some may not appreciate that they are being victimized. There may also be fear of repercussions from the trafficker when speaking up, or there may be distrust of health care providers or other authorities (Leslie 2018). Those experiencing exploitation have a lived perspective and perhaps a different understanding and definition of the nuances of their situation than services providers and researchers. It is vital to recognize this distinction.

In a study exploring commercial sexual exploitation of at-risk children (e.g., homeless, history of abuse) in Texas, the research team found a range of exploitative situations (Kellison et al. 2019). Alternatively, outside stakeholders often look for the "ideal" or "perfect" victim found at the nexus of the most severe vulnerabilities, risks, and acts of exploitation (Kellison et al. 2019). The majority of minors and youth who screened positively for commercial sexual exploitation also disclosed previous labor abuse or exploitation. This suggests that those economic drivers that led them to seek unsafe, less regulated, or informal work also contributed to their becoming sexually exploited (Kellison et al. 2019). Of note, the trafficked persons or respondents in this study were not asked about human trafficking or commercial sexual exploitation by their health care providers; rather, they were asked about their experiences with prior abuse, financial stability, support systems, and so on. In those discussions, several respondents then shared experiences—be it one or several sporadic periods of exploitation over years—when they were defrauded or coerced into trading sex for money or other needs, or when they had to trade sex as minors. That is to say, they largely did not identify with being "trafficked" or "engaging in commercial sex." The trafficking experiences occurred in the context of their vulnerable status (e.g., homelessness, violence, substance misuse, mental health issues, poverty). This is consistent with how perpetrators of violence take advantage of vulnerable individuals in order to gain control of their victims (Keeling and Fisher 2012). Figure 2–1 portrays these vulnerabilities as factors in becoming trafficked.

Although some tactics used by traffickers who exploit the vulnerabilities of minors and youth for commercial sex might differ from those who exploit adults and those who exploit other forms of labor, there will be similarities across all of these forms of violence. A pilot

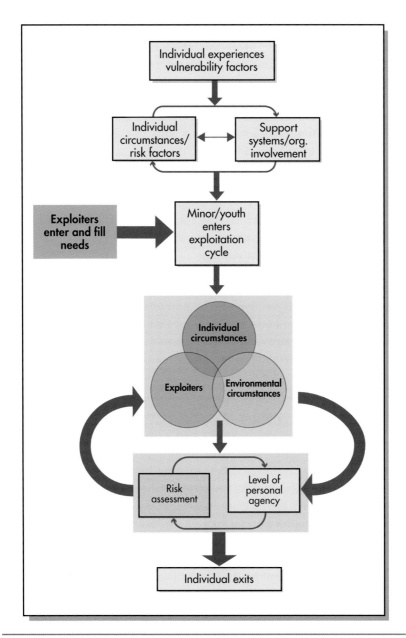

FIGURE 2–1. Concept map: life cycle of exploitation.

Source. Reprinted from Kellison B, Torres MIM, Kammer-Kerwick M, et al.: *"To the Public, Nothing Was Wrong With Me": Life Experiences of Minors and Youth in Texas at Risk for Commercial Sexual Exploitation.* Austin, TX, Institute on Domestic Violence and Sexual Assault, The University of Texas at Austin, 2019. Used with permission.

study exploring labor exploitation among immigrant laborers found that 11% of a laborer's time was exploited over their lifetime (Busch-Armendariz et al. 2016). Moreover, the laborers also did not identify as trafficking victims, nor did they or the research team use that language in discussing and detecting the exploitation (Busch-Armendariz et al. 2016). A survey of calls taken at a worker's center in Houston after Hurricane Harvey also explored the varying ways in which workers identified issues when they were seeking assistance with their experiences of exploitation (Acuña-Arreaza et al. 2019). In this study, the most common form of labor abuse was wage theft, which can range from not being offered the original hours promised to keeping someone in a work setting for an extended period of time without any pay. Figure 2–2 illustrates the range of exploitation experienced by the laborers calling in and their experiences with labor practices ranging from unjust to trafficking.

This pilot study and survey demonstrate again how important it is to adopt precise and validated definitions of human trafficking to understand the epidemiology of the problem. There are subtleties or nuances that extend beyond what may be portrayed in the media or what trafficked persons or health care providers may appreciate.

CONCLUSION

Knowing the epidemiology of human trafficking and its economic drivers is central to countering trafficking. Lessons learned from other prevention and harm reduction programs, especially those dealing with other forms of violence, could help to expand our understanding of the various forms of exploitation and to strengthen the effectiveness of identification, rehabilitation, and intervention efforts. A human rights perspective contributes to a broad conception of trafficking by emphasizing the individual's right to decent work, livable or fair wages, gender equality, and freedom from exploitation by force, fraud, or coercion. In this sense, public health and human rights go hand in hand, especially when considering the social determinants of health and systems of oppression that create inequalities in access to health care.

Pearls and Pointers

- To advocate for and support trafficked persons, a human rights perspective must be adopted.

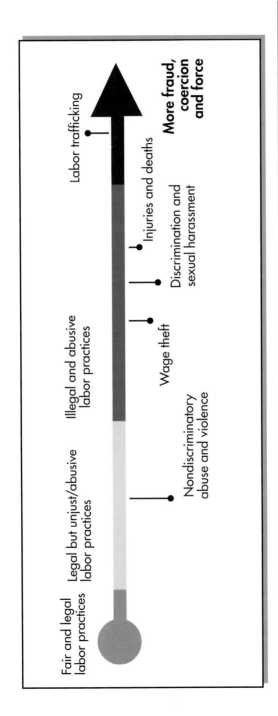

FIGURE 2–2. Spectrum of labor exploitation.

Source. Reprinted from Acuña-Arreaza M, Baldazo-Tudon K, Torres MIM: *A Year of Labor Abuse: A Visual Report of Rights Violations Faced by Houston Workers.* Houston, TX, Fe y Justicia Worker Center, 2019. Used with permission.

- Advocacy and human rights approaches should also identify and address systems of oppression that contribute to vulnerabilities for exploitation.

- Public health and human rights approaches do not merely state how to fight against human trafficking but also who should be engaged in these efforts.

- Human trafficking, as with other forms of violence, cannot be eradicated by rehabilitating victims alone; concerted intervention and prevention efforts are required.

REFERENCES

Acuña-Arreaza M, Baldazo-Tudon K, Torres MIM: A Year of Labor Abuse: A Visual Report of Rights Violations Faced by Houston Workers. Houston, TX, Fe y Justicia Worker Center, 2019

Busch-Armendariz NB, Nale NL, Kammer-Kerwick M, et al: Human Trafficking by the Numbers: The Initial Benchmark of Prevalence and Economic Impact for Texas. Austin, TX, Institute on Domestic Violence and Sexual Assault, The University of Texas at Austin, 2016

Decker MR: Sex trafficking, sex work, and violence: evidence for a new era. Int J Gynaecol Obstet 120(2):113–114, 2013 23228823

Falb KL, McCauley HL, Decker MR, et al: Trafficking mechanisms and HIV status among sex-trafficking survivors in Calcutta, India. Int J Gynaecol Obstet 113(1):86–87, 2011 21306708

Freire P: Pedagogy of the Oppressed (1970). Translated by Ramos MB. New York, Bloomsbury Academic, 2018

Hachtel H, Nixon M, Bennett D, et al: Motives, offending behavior, and gender differences in murder perpetrators with or without psychosis. J Interpers Violence :886260518774304, 2018 29759034

International Labour Organization: The prevention of occupational diseases. April 28, 2013. Available at: www.ilo.org/wcmsp5/groups/public/-
--ed_protect/---protrav/---safework/documents/publication/
wcms_208226.pdf. Accessed October 24, 2019.

International Labour Organization: Global estimates of modern slavery: forced labour and forced marriage. September 19, 2017. Available at: www.ilo.org/wcmsp5/groups/public/---dgreports/---dcomm/documents/
publication/wcms_575479.pdf. Accessed October 24, 2019.

Keeling J, Fisher C: Women's early relational experiences that lead to domestic violence. Qual Health Res 22(11):1559–1567, 2012 22910590

Kellison B, Torres MIM, Kammer-Kerwick M, et al: "To the public, nothing was wrong with me": life experiences of minors and youth in Texas at risk for commercial sexual exploitation. Institute on Domestic Violence and Sexual Assault, The University of Texas at Austin, March 2019. Available at: https://sites.utexas.edu/idvsa/files/2019/03/CSTT-HT-
Final-Report-3.26.19.pdf. Accessed October 23, 2019.

Kiss L, Zimmerman C: Human trafficking and labor exploitation: toward identifying, implementing, and evaluating effective responses. PLoS Med 16(1):e1002740, 2019 30695040

Kiss L, Pocock NS, Naisanguansri V, et al: Health of men, women, and children in post-trafficking services in Cambodia, Thailand, and Vietnam: an observational cross-sectional study. Lancet Glob Health 3(3):e154–e161, 2015 25701993

Leslie J: Human trafficking: clinical assessment guide. J Trauma Nurs 25(5):282–289, 2018 30216256

Lindhorst T, Tajima E: Reconceptualizing and operationalizing context in survey research on intimate partner violence. J Interpers Violence 23(3):362–388, 2008 18245573

Ngwe JE, Elechi OO: Human trafficking: the modern day slavery of the 21st century. African Journal of Criminology and Justice Studies 6(1/2):103–119, 2012

Panchanadeswaran S, Johnson SC, Sivaram S, et al: Intimate partner violence is as important as client violence in increasing street-based female sex workers' vulnerability to HIV in India. Int J Drug Policy 19(2):106–112, 2008 18187314

Polaris: The typology of modern slavery: defining sex and labor trafficking in the United States. March 2017. Available at: https://polarisproject.org/sites/default/files/Polaris-Typology-of-Modern-Slavery.pdf. Accessed October 24, 2019.

Reid JA: Entrapment and enmeshment schemes used by sex traffickers. Sex Abuse 28(6):491–511, 2016 25079777

Shadan KM: Human trafficking: modern day slavery in the 21st century. Canadian Foreign Policy 12(3):125–132, 2006

Sigmon JN: Combating modern-day slavery: issues in identifying and assisting victims of human trafficking worldwide. Victims and Offenders 3(2/3):245–257, 2008

Trafficking Victims Protection Act of 2000, Pub. L. No. 106-386 (22 U.S.C. § 7102). Available at: https://uscode.house.gov/view.xhtml?path=/prelim@title22/chapter78&edition=prelim. Accessed October 30, 2019.

Troshynski EI, Blank JK: Sex trafficking: an exploratory study interviewing traffickers. Trends Organ Crime 11(1):30–41, 2007

United Nations General Assembly: Universal declaration of human rights (217 [III] A). 1948. Available at: www.un.org/en/ga/search/view_doc.asp?symbol=A/RES/217(III). Accessed October 26, 2019.

United Nations General Assembly. Protocol against the smuggling of migrants by land, sea, and air, supplementing the United Nations Convention Against Transnational Organized Crime. 2000. Available at: www.unodc.org/documents/middleeastandnorthafrica/smuggling-migrants/SoM_Protocol_English.pdf. Accessed October 26, 2019.

United Nations General Assembly: Resolution adopted by the General Assembly on 25 September 2015: 70/1. Transforming our world: the 2030 agenda for sustainable development (A/RES/70/1; 25 September 2015). October 21, 2015. Available at: www.un.org/en/development/desa/population/migration/generalassembly/docs/globalcompact/A_RES_70_1_E.pdf. Accessed October 26, 2019.

U.S. Department of State: Trafficking in persons report. June 2017. Available at: www.state.gov/wp-content/uploads/2019/02/271339.pdf. Accessed October 24, 2019.

Walk Free Foundation: Global Slavery Index: United States. 2018. Available at: www.globalslaveryindex.org/2018/findings/country-studies/united-states/. Accessed October 23, 2019.

Weitzer R: New directions in research on human trafficking. Annals of the American Academy of Political Social Science 653(1):6–24, 2014

Wood SN, Glass N, Decker MR: An integrative review of safety strategies for women experiencing intimate partner violence in low- and middle-income countries. Trauma Violence Abuse 22:1524838018823270, 2019 30669943

World Health Organization: Global Health Observatory data repository: number of people (all ages) living with HIV—estimates by WHO region. November 7, 2018. Available at: http://apps.who.int/gho/data/view.main.22100WHO?lang=en. Accessed October 26, 2019.

World Health Organization, London School of Hygiene and Tropical Medicine, South African Medical Research Council: Global and regional estimates of violence against women: prevalence and health effects of intimate partner violence and non-partner sexual violence. 2013. Available at: https://apps.who.int/iris/bitstream/handle/10665/85239/9789241564625_eng.pdf;jsessionid=EB1AEFDB9A8A25106DFE162FD0B67BF0?sequence=1. Accessed October 26, 2019.

Zhang S: Measuring labor trafficking: a research note. Crime Law Soc Change 58(4):469–482, 2012

Zimmerman C, Kiss L: Human trafficking and exploitation: a global health concern. PLoS Medicine 14(11):e1002437, 2017 29166396

CHAPTER 3

By the Right Name

WHAT DOES IT ACTUALLY MEAN TO
"SCREEN" AND "ASSESS" FOR
TRAFFICKING IN HEALTH CARE?

Makini Chisolm-Straker, M.D., M.P.H.

> The beginning of wisdom is to call things by their
> proper name.
> —*Confucius*

A middle-aged man presents to the emergency department for flank pain that radiates to the right side of his abdomen. He has had the pain for 1 day, but it is excruciating. Sometimes the pain is so overwhelming he vomits. He has tried acetaminophen but has felt no relief. At triage, the nurse runs through the barrage of required questions, although it's obvious the patient has a kidney stone. "Have you traveled outside the country in the past month?" "No." "Do you want a free HIV test?" "OK." "Have you been hit, kicked, punched, or otherwise hurt by someone in the past year?" "Um, yes." The nurse raises an eyebrow and looks from the computer screen to the patient. "Oh, OK. I will get the social worker." Fast forward, and I see this patient in the clinic where I volunteer. There I learned that he was forced to shoplift to have the items resold on the street. Failure to comply resulted in beatings and threats of arrest for criminal activity. He came to the emergency department for a kidney stone, and he left with a real connection to services that allowed him and his children a "new lease on life."

THE BEGINNING OF WISDOM

Since the American Public Health Association's policy statement on human trafficking in 2015 and the federal government's acceptance in

2016 of the conceptualization of human trafficking as a public health problem, labor and sex trafficking has been more commonly regarded as "not just a crime" (American Public Health Association 2015; Chon 2016). Convenience sampling data indicate that people present to health care settings during their trafficking experience, and their situations are often unrecognized by the clinical care team (Baldwin et al. 2011; Chisolm-Straker et al. 2016; Lederer and Wetzel 2014). Increasingly, states are requiring that clinicians receive training on the topic, and in 2015, the federal government made clinicians mandated reporters for concerns of trafficking of minors (Atkinson et al. 2016; Child Abuse Prevention and Treatment Act (P.L. 155-271). In the talk about how clinicians can serve this patient population, the terms *screening, assessment,* and *response protocol* are often heard. These terms are often used incorrectly and interchangeably. If language use indicates clinician action, term confusion can imperil the safety and care of the patients whom clinicians aim to serve. To improve the clinical care of previously unrecognized persons who have experienced trafficking, a clarity of vocabulary is prudent. In this chapter, the reader will learn the clinical difference between *screening, assessment,* and *protocols* and the limitations of current screening and assessment instruments. In this chapter, terms are defined with respect to their clinical application, and their utility in the public health–framed anti-trafficking movement is elucidated. See Table 3–1 for the definition of terms that will be used throughout this chapter.

SCREENING

General Principles

A screening tool systematically allows for testing of an entire group for the possible presence of an outcome of interest; its purpose is to determine whether someone needs assessment for the outcome of interest (Maxim et al. 2014; Stoto et al. 1999; Substance Abuse and Mental Health Services Administration 2009). The instrument should be applied to an at-risk population, *regardless* of the user's suspicion for the outcome of interest. This allows those with the outcome of interest to be identified regardless of the tester's biases or subjective judgments. In the clinical example at the start of this chapter, the triage nurse asked a validated (see Table 3–1) intimate partner violence screening question even though the diagnosis for

TABLE 3–1.   Terms used in the treatment of trafficked persons

TERM	DEFINITION
Human trafficking	The recruitment, harboring, transportation, provision, and/or obtaining of a person by the use of force, fraud, and/or coercion, for the purposes of labor and/or sexual exploitation. In the case of minors (under the age of 18 years), third-party facilitation is not needed for a determination of sex trafficking; minor involvement in any kind of commercial sexual activity meets the federal definition of human trafficking (Trafficking Victims Protection Act of 2000; P.L. 106-386).
Clinician/ practitioner	A health care practitioner qualified to provide, and in the practice of providing, mental and/or medical health services to patients. For the purposes of this chapter, such persons may be physician assistants, nurse practitioners, physicians, psychologists, social workers, or counselors.
Trafficked person	A person with an experience (current or past) of labor and/or sex trafficking. (The author purposefully declines to use the term *victim* in reference to people with a trafficking experience, as this is law enforcement terminology and not relevant to clinical care. Furthermore, the author recognizes the survivorship of people in the midst of a trafficking situation and that the experience of trafficking is not a "one off" for many [i.e., people may experience trafficking situations multiple times]. And although *survivor* can be applied to anyone with a trafficking experience [regardless of whether they are in or out of their situation], it is often presumed to mean those no longer in their situation. In this chapter, *survivor* is only used to refer to people no longer in a trafficking situation.)
Screening	The simple testing of all members of a particular population for a specific outcome of interest. The outcome of a screen is dichotomous; it is positive or negative. A positive screen is not necessarily diagnostic, but it identifies individuals who need further assessment.

TABLE 3-1. Terms used in the treatment of trafficked persons *(continued)*

TERM	DEFINITION
Assessment	An expert evaluation of a person used in the setting of concern for an outcome of interest. The concern may stem from the expertise of a proficient clinician or a positive screen.
Protocol	An algorithmic action plan enacted when an outcome or potential for an outcome is appreciated and warrants response from a team.
Validation	Confirmation that the tool measures what it claims to measure, among those for whom it is employed.
Sensitivity	A test's capacity to identify the outcome of interest.
Specificity	A test's capacity to exclude, or rule out, the presence of the outcome of interest.
Multidisciplinary	An approach that meaningfully involves patients/clients and professionals from multiple, relevant disciplines working together toward a common goal. Team members can be from multiple institutions and agencies and do not need to be health care based.
Trauma-informed care	Care that promotes resilience in patients, clinicians, and all care team members; this approach encourages all parties to actively work to avoid retraumatization or triggered decline into distress.
Patient-centered care	Care plans that are collaboratively developed with the patient so that the patient's goals and needs are purposefully placed at the forefront of all clinical decisions.

Note. Terms are listed in the order in which they appear in the chapter text.

the chief complaint seemed obvious to the nurse. In this way, the nurse allowed the patient the opportunity to disclose more history that was not immediately or discernibly relevant to his probable kidney stone but certainly had an impact on his overall well-being.

Ideally, a screening tool is short and does not require particular expertise to administer or interpret. The delineation, or cutoff, between a positive or negative screen is predetermined and clear prior to use. In this way, an instrument can be quickly but consistently applied to a large group of people and can facilitate identification of people with or at high risk for the outcome of interest.

Validated Trafficking Screening Tool Examples

Short Screen for Child Sex Trafficking

The Short Screen for Child Sex Trafficking (SSCST) is the first (and at the time of this writing, the only) validated trafficking screening tool for use in the health care setting (Kaltiso et al. 2018). It is a screening tool in that it is short, simple to administer, highly sensitive (90.9%), and does not require expert interpretation. However, it does benefit from expert application, as it is only applied to specific chief complaints or when the clinician is concerned about trafficking (more akin to an assessment; see the "Assessment" section). Of note, this instrument is not comprehensive; it only enables screening for child sex trafficking among certain 13- to 17-year-old English-speaking patients.

Quick Youth Indicators for Trafficking

Quick Youth Indicators for Trafficking (QYIT) meets the ideal definition of a screening tool, in that it is short, does not require expert administration or interpretation, and has high sensitivity (86.7%). This screening tool has only been validated for use only among homeless young adults receiving social services, *not* in the health care setting (Chisolm-Straker et al. 2019).

Multiple institutions, organizations, and agencies use various other trafficking screening tools. For example, the National Human Trafficking Training and Technical Assistance Center (NHTTAC) has developed a tool for clinicians to screen for labor and sex trafficking in adult patients (Administration for Children and Families, Office on Trafficking in Persons, and the National Human Trafficking Training and Technical Assistance Center 2018). Most "screening tools" focus on sex trafficking and/or, like the NHTTAC tool, are not validated (Armstrong 2017; Bespalova et al. 2016). This limits their applicability and may bias conclusions made about subjects who are screened or understandings about trafficking at a population level.

ASSESSMENT

General Principles

An assessment may be employed when there is already concern for an outcome of interest; it is implemented when a proficient user recognizes potential for utility (Maxim et al. 2014; Stoto et al. 1999; Substance Abuse and Mental Health Services Administration 2009). Apt use of an assessment instrument relies on the expertise of the user and calls for purposeful application of resources. For example, among patients with chest pain, only those with specific historical risk factors or exam findings are assessed, via blood tests and/or imaging, for a pulmonary embolism (Kline 2018; Penaloza et al. 2017). In this way, other patients with chest pain avoid expensive, time-consuming, and/or risky testing.

Validated Trafficking Assessment Tool Examples

Trafficking Victim Identification Tool

The Vera Institute's Trafficking Victim Identification Tool (TVIT) was the first validated "screening" tool for human trafficking; however, because it requires expert interpretation, it is discussed here as an example of an assessment (Simich et al. 2014).

Human Trafficking Identification Assessment Measure–14

The Human Trafficking Identification Assessment Measure–14 (HTIAM-14) is a trafficking assessment tool that was developed based on the TVIT (Bigelsen and Vuotto 2013). It is somewhat shorter and can also be applied to an entire population (e.g., homeless youth receiving social services), but, like the TVIT, it requires expert interpretation.

These are two validated, structured trafficking assessments; however, trafficking assessments do not have to be structured. For example, the TVIT was tested in a variety of ways, including comparison to the trafficking determination of immigration lawyers and social workers with trafficking service expertise (Simich et al. 2014). The example assessments above, although validated, are not appropriate for the health care setting: they have not been validated in a patient population, and given the length of time required to administer and the expertise needed to interpret the results, they are too onerous for clinical use. That is to say, in the course of routine and emergency health care, most clinicians do not usually have an additional 45–60 minutes to perform these assessments for each patient. Furthermore, most health care practitioners are not experts in human trafficking and thus should not be interpreting the results of the assessment.

As with available trafficking screening instruments, there are a multitude of other trafficking assessment tools. For example, Polaris's assessment tool is intended to help users assess for labor and/ or sex trafficking (Polaris 2011). But at the time of this writing, most assessments, like that of Polaris, are also unvalidated and not designed for use in the health care setting.

VALIDATION

Validation of a screening or assessment tool indicates that the instrument tests or measures what it purports to test or measure and is appropriate for a particular setting and/or population (Figure 3–1). Acceptable, high-quality validation means that the new instrument has been compared with a logical or gold standard, and the gold standard is considered conclusive (Greenhalgh 1997; Maxim et al. 2014). An example of testing against a gold standard would be comparing a novel test's capacity to identify a pulmonary embolism with the performance of a computed tomographic angiography for a pulmonary embolism. The work of Brucker et al. (2018) in testing the use of a suicidality screening tool exemplifies the use of a logical standard: the team tested the screening tool against patient report of suicide attempt at 6 months.

Screening instruments and structured assessments that are built and founded solely on expert opinion or recommendation are *not* validated, because they are not strictly empirically based. Even well-informed opinions do not always accurately reflect reality and are subject to the biases of the opinion holders. Unvalidated screening tools are, at best, unvalidated assessment tools, because they rely on opinion (expert or otherwise) rather than empirical evidence. Reliance on opinion for instrument development biases collection of data (and thus understanding of the outcome of interest) at a population level and clinical care at the individual level.

In a clinical setting, if an instrument purports to measure something but actually measures something else, use by clinicians may harm an individual and/or a population. For example, if a urine test is *thought* to test for pregnancy but *actually* tests for cancer, a person may reasonably assume a positive result means they are pregnant and will not seek curative or palliative care for cancer.[1] Delay in the cancer diagnosis may result in loss of life or decreased quality of life.

---

[1]Because traditionally, Western gendered pronouns exclude gender nonconforming or "genderqueer" individuals, the chapter author uses plural pronouns in lieu of singular, dichotomously gendered ones.

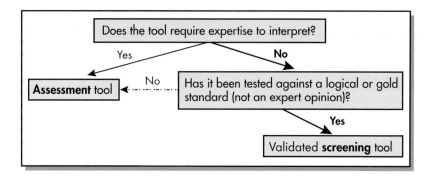

FIGURE 3–1. Understanding trafficking evaluation tools.

Similarly, when instruments purport to test for human trafficking but actually only test for one type of trafficking, instrument users do a disservice to those who are tested. Many human trafficking screening tests only test for, or are biased in favor of finding, sex trafficking experiences. For those who test "negative" for trafficking on such instruments, "negative" may only pertain to sex trafficking. This means that those with a labor trafficking experience who test "negative" may not receive the opportunity to seek services specific to their labor trafficking situation(s). Moreover, communities will systematically underrecognize labor trafficking and consequently (continue to) not provide sufficient resources for labor trafficking prevention and intervention.

It is also important to examine a screening test for the validity of its use in particular populations and settings. For example, the Convergent Functional Information for Suicidality Scale (CFI-S) has proven useful for predicting suicidality in psychiatric patients, but, until the work of the Brucker et al. 2018 group, it had not been tested for application in the general emergency department setting/patient population. A test may perform well in one setting or group but not in another for a variety of reasons. For example, if the test is long or cumbersome, respondents in some settings may not have the time to complete the test. If the test is written, use in a nonliterate or low-literacy population may alter its performance. If the test has not been trialed in various languages, it may underidentify or overidentify the outcome of interest when applied to people who use a language other than that in which the tool was designed/tested. Or the populations used for tool development and the populations actually being screened may be inherently different. One group may be at higher risk for an outcome, such that use of the screening instrument is inappropriate; it may be that the group at increased risk should receive an in-depth assessment or intervention rather than a screening. Here again, we return to the pulmonary embolism example. The D-dimer test is useful in patients with chest pain who have a low probability of having pulmonary embolism as their diagnosis. If the patient is at high risk of having a pulmonary embolism, a D-dimer test (as a screening test) is an inappropriate evaluation, and an imaging assessment is warranted.

Clinicians recognize the import of using validated tools in other aspects of clinical care, and patients with a trafficking experience deserve those same high standards. Validated tools for trafficking identification exist, but at the time of this writing, the SSCST is the only one that is validated for the clinical care setting (Kaltiso et al. 2018). Yet, as noted in the discussion of the SSCST, it is limited in that it only screens for sex trafficking among those ages 13–17 years.

SENSITIVITY AND SPECIFICITY

In addition to being valid, a screening tool must be highly sensitive. *Sensitivity* refers to a test's capacity to identify the outcome of interest; *specificity* refers to a test's capacity to exclude, or rule out, the outcome of interest. To allow the user to identify the outcome of interest, a good screening instrument values sensitivity over specificity. A screening instrument with high sensitivity will have few *false negatives*—results identifying people who truly have the outcome of interest but test negative. The goal is to have as few false negatives as possible so that those with the outcome of interest can receive appropriate interventions. If the test has not been validated, however, its "sensitivity" is much less meaningful because the test is not known to capture the outcome of interest.

A specificity that is too low will produce many *false positives*—results identifying people without the outcome of interest but who test positive. Such persons will require further testing or may inappropriately receive interventions. A very low (or bad) specificity may result in an overburdened system via inappropriate resource allocation, in (possibly risky) assessments of the people that screened falsely positive, in unnecessary and/or harmful interventions, and in undue fear in the individuals who falsely test positive.

To better grasp the application of sensitivity and specificity principles, consider the standard urine pregnancy test. This validated screening test is available for use by laypersons because it does not require expertise or significant training to use and interpret. The urine pregnancy test is highly sensitive, so it will identify most (98%) pregnancies 7 days after implantation (Chard 1992). In a clinical setting, this test is a very good way to exclude an ectopic pregnancy as a cause for abdominal pain in cisgender women.[2] The urine pregnancy test also has a good specificity, so most people who are not pregnant will test negative. Furthermore, the test is highly *reliable*, meaning it will produce consistent results in the same person, with repeated correct use.

To be sensitive a tool must be validated against a gold or logical standard. For example, the SSCST is highly sensitive (90.9%) for its intended population; the SSCST was validated against an internationally recognized expert assessment (logical standard). This tells the user that when used appropriately, the SSCST is very good at identifying pediatric patients (ages 13–17 years) who should be assessed by an expert for sex trafficking experiences. (Remember, a positive screening outcome is *not* necessarily diagnostic.)

DISCLOSURE CAVEATS

Screening and Assessment "Success"

Clinical screening and assessments aim to identify an outcome so that health care practitioners can offer intervention. The primary focus of clinical care must always be high-quality, evidence-based (whenever possible) care to those in need. Clinicians in various settings routinely screen for outcomes commonly recognized as falling within the health spectrum, such as pregnancy, diabetes, depression, and alcohol use disorder. However, under legal mandate, social problems (which also impact health) such as child maltreatment, elder abuse, intimate partner violence, and now human trafficking also falls within our purview.

To be clear, the clinician's job is not to *investigate* for these issues—that is why reports are made—but to facilitate patients' connection to needed services. The Child Abuse Prevention and Treatment Act (P.L. 155-271) now mandates clinician report of suspicion of labor or sex trafficking of minors, but not all states require reports to their central registries or law enforcement. States vary regarding which

---

[2]Persons whose affirmed gender is the same as that which was assigned/assumed at birth, not transgender or gender nonconforming.

legal entity must receive such reports (e.g., child maltreatment registries versus law enforcement). Practitioners must familiarize themselves with the laws of the state(s) in which they practice.

Clinical recognition of trafficking requires that 1) the screening and/or assessment be conducted in an environment hospitable to disclosure and 2) the subject be ready to disclose. Unlike a pregnancy test, which is either objectively positive or negative, a trafficking screen or assessment can be positive or negative based on the patient's conception of their situation, the patient's understanding of the questions, the interpretation of the results by the person administering the instrument (assessment only), the patient's comfort in sharing information with the person asking, or any number of other factors. A successful screening or assessment is not necessarily one in which a clinician "achieves" disclosure, but it is one in which the patient believes that disclosure would be safe and useful. Other chapters in this book offer types of questions individual clinicians have found useful in respectfully asking about patient experiences with interpersonal violence generally and possible trafficking specifically.

Special Populations and Clinical Implications

The screening and assessment tools highlighted in this chapter were all conducted among medically and psychologically stable, mature persons (clients or patients) with the capacity to participate. However, case reports, expert opinion, and convenience sample data indicate that having intellectual developmental disorder (IDD) and/or mental illness increases the risk of being trafficked (Chisolm-Straker et al. 2018; Hawkins 2017; Institute of Medicine and National Research Council 2013; Nguyen et al. 2018; *United States v. Callahan* 2015; *United States v. Kozminski* 1988). It is unknown how instruments will perform in those with IDD or mental illness because the instruments were not tested or validated in these populations. Thus, it is not known whether these instruments will underidentify or overidentify (if either) labor and/or sex trafficking in these groups. This means that clinicians should not accept the "outcomes" of these screenings and assessments at face value especially when administered in these groups.

Clinicians must *always* be ready to accept a disclosure and must cultivate an environment conducive to disclosure, even when a screen or assessment was previously negative. This is certainly true of clinicians who have longer relationships with patients, throughout the life course, because patients may not be trafficked at the time of first screening or assessment but may be later in life. Or the patient may be more comfortable sharing when a trusting, professional care relationship has been cultivated. In persons with IDD and mental illness, clinicians should purposefully and systematically revisit the possibility of a trafficking experience (Nguyen et al. 2018). In patients with exacerbated or untreated mental illness, clinicians should not dismiss reported experiences because they are shared during a period when the patient's illness is exacerbated. Disclosures can be revisited if the patient (re)gains the capacity to meaningfully participate in providing a history (patient's capacity to comprehend instrument questions and/or recall life events may improve) and to understand the ramifications of disclosure (including patients who are younger than 18 years). Clinicians should remember to pose screening and assessment questions at a pace that patients can absorb. And although the language used should be true to the validated instrument, explanations may be required to help patients with IDD or a low literacy level understand the intent of the question.

For patients who do not demonstrate capacity, disclosures should still be seriously considered because this group may be particularly vulnerable to exploitation and abuse. Serious considerations entail mandated reporting when appropriate (e.g., minors) and connection to needed services if clinically relevant.

BEYOND SCREENING AND/OR ASSESSMENT

Ethical Considerations and Patient-Centered Care

Systematic screening or assessment for human trafficking is irresponsible in the absence of institutional capacity to connect affected patients with relevant services (if the patient desires). Health care institutions should develop robust human trafficking response protocols prior to enacting systematic human trafficking evaluation (screening or assessment). Without institutional support, clinicians with trafficking expertise may consider asking about possible trafficking situations but should be prepared to 1) report to appropriate agencies when relevant (e.g., minors) and 2) actively support patients in the connection to services. Asking but subsequently doing nothing to support patient disclosures is unethical.

At the time of this writing, there are no comprehensive (labor and sex trafficking) validated screening tools for use in the clinical setting, and all health care practitioners cannot become experts in human trafficking assessment. Thus, institutions should focus on training clinicians to be competent to consider human trafficking (similar to clinicians' child maltreatment awareness) and on developing locally relevant institutional response protocols.

Part of such education teaches practitioners to employ patient-centered and trauma-informed techniques (behaviors and manners of speech) in routine care. Such education teaches practitioners to conceive of a patient as a whole person, not only a pathologized body and/or mind. For example, clinicians may learn to ask about patients' plans to return to work or how an illness or injury will impact their ability to work. A clearly clinically relevant question allows for a natural opportunity for clinicians to open a dialog about a patient's social milieu and safety outside of the health care facility. (For more on the trauma-informed, patient-centered clinical approach, see Chapter 8, "Responding to Trafficked Persons in Health Care Settings.")

Protocol

A *protocol* is a detailed plan of procedure (Merriam-Webster 2019). A protocol is enacted when an outcome or potential for an outcome is appreciated and warrants response. Pertinent activation of a protocol mobilizes a dedicated set of team members and/or assets when an outcome, or concern for an outcome, arises. For example, when a mandated reporter suspects child maltreatment, a protocol may help determine if the concern is meritorious, what other professionals should be enlisted to investigate and respond, and what are the next steps in care and intervention.

Multiple health care institutions, organizations, and agencies have human trafficking concern and/or recognition response protocols. Stoklosa et al. (2017) reviewed 30 protocols of health care institutions from 19 states and two professional organizations in the United States. The team explored many items of protocol inclusion, such as how many protocols defined human trafficking, provided examples of indicators of trafficking, explained mandatory reporting laws, or included referral and resource contact information. Given the breadth and depth of that review article, further discussion of protocols is not warranted at the time of this writing. Interested readers should refer to the article by Stoklosa and colleagues. For guidance on developing a multidisciplinary (including survivors), trauma-in-

formed, patient-centered protocol, readers can refer to the protocol
tool kit developed by HEAL Trafficking and Hope for Justice (HEAL
Trafficking and Hope for Justice 2017).

CONCLUSION

More data are needed to determine the populations for whom systematic screening for labor and/or sex trafficking is appropriate and
the patient impact of such screenings. Well-intentioned clinician efforts to "identify" trafficking can be harmful to patients if clinicians
aggressively attempt to uncover victimizations and "rescue" patients.
Although legal authorities may conceptualize trafficking as a crime,
not all people whose experiences meet the federal definition identify
as victimized (Anahita 2000; Connor 2016; Goździak 2016; Walters
2019; Young Women's Empowerment Project 2009). Practitioners
should provide evidence-based, comprehensive, accessible, and compassionate health care. Practitioners must also be patient: human
trafficking is complex and a centuries-old problem. To improve care
of this patient population, institutions and clinicians should take
survivor-informed, science-based actions rather than only relying on
implicit biases about how "victims" and "perpetrators" present.
Lacking comprehensive, validated screening and assessment tools
for use in the health care setting, for now, health care practitioners
can do for trafficking as we should do for other forms of interpersonal
violence for which we lack such instruments. Institutions can employ systematic comprehensive training, and clinicians can routinely
(with all patients) use a patient-centered and trauma-informed care
approach and rely on multidisciplinary teams when anti-trafficking
protocol activation is clinically germane.

Pearls and Pointers

- Screening focuses on an entire, predetermined population for an outcome of interest. A good screening test is
  brief, has a high sensitivity, and has been validated for
  use in a particular population and setting.

- Assessment is performed by a topical expert and is conducted based on expert judgment and/or a positive
  screening.

- There are major gaps in the trafficking screening tools
  currently in existence. In particular, most trafficking

screening tools are unvalidated and/or only screen for sex trafficking.

- Using validated tools to screen for trafficking more equitably allows for patient disclosure.

- Given the present lack of comprehensive, validated screening tools, clinician training on labor and sex trafficking is essential. With comprehensive, systematic education, practitioners will know when and how to respectfully probe when there is a clinical concern for trafficking.

- Aggressive clinician effort to obtain disclosure of a trafficking experience can be harmful to patients. Pressuring patients to share what they do not want or are not ready to share is disrespectful and injurious to the patient-practitioner relationship. Moreover, clinician focus on one outcome may result in failure to allow a patient to share about another experience or situation. Health care practitioners should use a trauma-informed, patient-centered approach to care interactions to allow patients the space to disclose if and when they are ready (see Chapter 8).

- Institutions should not engage in systematic screening without the capacity to assess and provide services, or refer for assessment and service provision. Development of a multidisciplinary (including survivors), trauma-informed, patient-centered response protocol prior to systematic efforts to recognize trafficking among a patient population is ethically responsible. These protocols enable clinicians to more readily connect patients to community-based anti-trafficking organizations that can offer trafficked persons more complete support than health care alone. Responsible protocol development is available at low cost, and many successful models already exist.

REFERENCES

Administration for Children and Families, Office on Trafficking in Persons, and the National Human Trafficking Training and Technical Assistance Center: Adult human trafficking screening tool and guide. 2018. Available at: www.acf.hhs.gov/sites/default/files/otip/adult_human_trafficking_screening_tool_and_guide.pdf. Accessed October 29, 2019.

American Public Health Association: Expanding and coordinating human trafficking-related public health research, evaluation, education, and prevention. Policy Number 201516. 2015. Available at: www.apha.org/policies-and-advocacy/public-health-policy-statements/policy-database/2016/01/26/14/28/expanding-and-coordinating-human-trafficking-related-public-health-activities. Accessed October 29, 2019.

Anahita JM: Dancing on shaky ground: the power-laden interactions between exotic dancers and their customers. Retrospective Theses and Dissertations, 16802. 2000. Available at: http://lib.dr.iastate.edu/cgi/viewcontent.cgi?article=17801&context=rtd. Accessed October 29, 2019.

Armstrong S: Instruments to identify commercially sexually exploited children: feasibility of use in an emergency department setting. Pediatr Emerg Care 33(12):794–799, 2017 28072670

Atkinson HG, Curnin KJ, Hanson NC: U.S. state laws addressing human trafficking: education of and mandatory reporting by health care providers and other professionals. Journal of Human Trafficking 2(2):111–138, 2016

Baldwin SB, Eisenman DP, Sayles JN, et al: Identification of human trafficking victims in health care settings. Health Hum Rights 13(1):E36–E49, 2011 22772961

Bespalova N, Morgan J, Coverdale J: A pathway to freedom: an evaluation of screening tools for the identification of trafficking victims. Acad Psychiatry 40(1):124–128, 2016 25398267

Bigelsen J, Vuotto S: Homelessness, survival sex, and human trafficking: as experienced by the youth of Covenant House New York. Covenant House, May 2013. Available at: https://humantraffickinghotline.org/sites/default/files/Homelessness%2C%20Survival%20Sex%2C%20and%20Human%20Trafficking%20-%20Covenant%20House%20NY.pdf. Accessed October 28, 2019.

Brucker K, Duggan C, Niezer J, et al: Assessing risk of future suicidality in emergency department patients. Acad Emerg Med 26(4):376–383, 2019 30375082

Chard T: Pregnancy tests: a review. Hum Reprod 7(5):701–710, 1992 1639991

Child Abuse Prevention and Treatment Act (as amended by P.L. 155-271), 132 STAT 3894, October 24, 2018

Chisolm-Straker M, Baldwin S, Gaïgbé-Togbé B, et al: Health care and human trafficking: we are seeing the unseen. J Health Care Poor Underserved 27(3):1220–1233, 2016 27524764

Chisolm-Straker M, Sze J, Einbond J, et al: A supportive adult may be the difference in homeless youth not being trafficked. Child Youth Serv Rev 91:115–120, 2018

Chisolm-Straker M, Sze J, Einbond J, et al: Screening for human trafficking among homeless young adults. Child Youth Serv Rev 98:72–79, 2019

Chon K: The power of framing human trafficking as public health issue. Office on Trafficking in Persons. 2016. Available at: www.acf.hhs.gov/otip/resource/publichealthlens. Accessed October 29, 2019.

Connor BM: In loco aequitatis: the dangers of "safe harbor" laws for youth in the sex trades. Stanford Journal of Civil Rights and Civil Liberties 12(43):45–116, 2016

Goździak EM: Forced victims or willing migrants? Contesting assumptions about child trafficking, in Contested Childhoods: Growing up in Migrancy. IMISCOE Research Series. Edited by Seeberg M, Goździak E. Cham, Switzerland, Springer, 2016, pp 23–41

Greenhalgh T: How to read a paper. Papers that report diagnostic or screening tests. BMJ 315(7107):540–543, 1997 9329312

Hawkins D: White restaurant manager enslaved black man for years, federal prosecutors say. The Washington Post, October 12, 2017. Available at: www.washingtonpost.com/news/morning-mix/wp/2017/10/12/white-restaurant-manager-enslaved-black-man-for-years-federal-prosecutors-say/?noredirect=on. Accessed October 29, 2019.

HEAL Trafficking, Hope for Justice: HEAL Trafficking and Hope for Justice's Protocol Toolkit. 2017. Available at: https://healtrafficking.org/2017/06/new-heal-trafficking-and-hope-for-justices-protocol-toolkit-for-developing-a-response-to-victims-of-human-trafficking-in-health-care-settings/. Accessed October 29, 2019.

Institute of Medicine, National Research Council: Confronting Commercial Sexual Exploitation and Sex Trafficking of Minors in the United States. Washington, DC, National Academies Press, 2013

Kaltiso SO, Greenbaum VJ, Agarwal M, et al: Evaluation of a screening tool for child sex trafficking among patients with high-risk chief complaints in a pediatric emergency department. Acad Emerg Med 25(11):1193–1203, 2018 30381877

Kline JA: Diagnosis and exclusion of pulmonary embolism. Thromb Res 163:207–220, 2018 28683951

Lederer LJ, Wetzel CA: The health consequences of sex trafficking and their implications for identifying victims in healthcare facilities. Annals of Health Law 23(1):61–87, 2014

Maxim LD, Niebo R, Utell MJ: Screening tests: a review with examples. Inhal Toxicol 26(13):811–828, 2014 25264934

Merriam-Webster: Protocol. 2019. Available at: www.merriam-webster.com/dictionary/protocol. Accessed October 29, 2019.

Nguyen PT, Lamkin J, Coverdale JH, et al: Identifying human trafficking victims on a psychiatry inpatient service: a case series. Psychiatr Q 89(2):341–348, 2018 28971296

Penaloza A, Soulié C, Moumneh T, et al: Pulmonary embolism rule-out criteria (PERC) rule in European patients with low implicit clinical probability (PERCEPIC): a multicentre, prospective, observational study. Lancet Haematol 4(12):e615–e621, 2017 28971296

Polaris: Comprehensive human trafficking assessment. 2011. Available at: https://humantraffickinghotline.org/sites/default/files/Comprehensive%20Trafficking%20Assessment.pdf. Accessed October 28, 2019.

Simich L, Goyen L, Powell A, et al: Improving human trafficking victim identification—validation and dissemination of a screening tool. Vera Institute of Justice, 2014. Available at: www.ncjrs.gov/pdffiles1/nij/grants/246713.pdf. Accessed October 29, 2019.

Stoklosa H, Dawson MB, Williams-Oni F, et al: A review of U.S. health care institution protocols for the identification and treatment of victims of human trafficking. Journal of Human Trafficking 3(2):116–124, 2017

Stoto MA, Almario DA, McCormick MC (eds): Reducing the Odds: Preventing Perinatal Transmission of HIV in the United States. Institute of Medicine, Committee on Perinatal Transmission of HIV. Washington, DC, National Academies Press, 1999

Substance Abuse and Mental Health Services Administration: Chapter 4: Screening and Assessment, in Substance Abuse Treatment: Addressing the Specific Needs of Women. Treatment Improvement Protocol (TIP) Series, No 51. Center for Substance Abuse Treatment, 2009. Available at: www.ncbi.nlm.nih.gov/books/NBK83253/. Accessed October 29, 2019.

United States v Callahan, Nos. 14-3771, 14-3772 (6th Cir. Sept. 8, 2015)

United States v Kozminski, 487 U.S. 921 (1988)

Trafficking Victims Protection Act of, Pub. L. No. 106-386; reauthorized by the Trafficking Victims Protection Reauthorization Act (TVPRA) of, Pub. L. No. 108-193; the TVPRA of, Pub. L. No. 109-164; and the William Wilberforce Trafficking Victims Protection Reauthorization Act (WW-TVPA) of, Pub. L. No. 110-457; and the TVPRA of 2013, Pub. L. No. 113-114

Walters K: The problem with forced rescue and detention in anti-trafficking initiatives. Alliance, February 28, 2019. Available at: https://delta87.org/2019/02/problem-forced-rescue-and-detention-anti-trafficking-initiatives/. Accessed October 29, 2019.

Young Women's Empowerment Project: Girls do what they have to do to survive: illuminating methods used by girls in the sex trade and street economy to fight back and heal. 2009. Available at: https://ywep-chicago.files.wordpress.com/2011/06/girls-do-what-they-have-to-do-to-survive-a-study-of-resilience-and-resistance.pdf. Accessed October 29, 2019.

CHAPTER 4

Barriers to Identification of Trafficked Persons in Health Care Settings

Frances Recknor, L.C.S.W., Dr.P.H.

Hanni Stoklosa, M.D., M.P.H.

Cathy L. Miller, R.N., Ph.D.

> We cannot rely upon the silenced to tell us they are suffering.
>
> —*Hanan Ashrawi, Palestinian leader, legislator, and activist*

This was Jorge's first time in an emergency department. He only came because he had to. He cut off his thumb while sawing some boards for a construction job he was working on. He didn't speak English and declined an interpreter. The hand surgeon evaluated him and said that they could attempt to reattach his thumb, but he would need to take time off from work. Jorge wanted the bleeding to stop and to be able to go back to work as soon as possible. After all, he had incurred a huge debt in order to come to the United States and was being paid very little. If he stopped working, for even a day, he feared that family in his home country might be harmed. He was discharged home on antibiotics and told to follow up in the hand clinic 1 week later. Jorge was "lost to follow-up."

Jorge's story reflects what might be a common occurrence for trafficked individuals who seek health and mental health care. Jorge came and left without anyone realizing the true nature of the circumstances under which he sustained his traumatic injury—he was a trafficked laborer. Language and cultural barriers inhibited thoughtful discussion between Jorge and his health care provider (HCP) as no interpreter was present. Furthermore, Jorge may not have realized that the conditions under which he worked in the United States were considered exploitative. He was not aware that he had rights as a worker, so he did not know he could receive assistance if he asked for it. All Jorge knew was that he could not take more time off from work, even if it meant losing his thumb. He feared that the trafficker would take retribution on his family if he stopped working. As a result of circumstantial confluence, Jorge did not receive a treatment plan tailored to his trafficking predicament; he did not have the opportunity to discuss his situation with someone who might be able to refer him to resources for assistance or to help him to leave his trafficker if this was what he wished. Jorge never returned to a provider for his injury and an opportunity to assist him with his circumstances was missed.

Jorge's story illustrates how HCPs are well positioned to identify and intervene with patients who have been trafficked for labor and/or commercial sexual exploitation. Moreover, studies show that an HCP may be one of few professionals who encounter trafficked persons while they are being exploited (Chisolm-Straker et al. 2016). Research also reflects that trafficked persons may exhibit a complex mixture of adverse acute and chronic mental and physical health outcomes. Adverse mental health outcomes may include anxiety, depression, substance use disorders, self-harm behaviors, and suicidal ideation (Powell et al. 2018). Physical health outcomes may include HIV and other sexually transmitted infections, gastrointestinal issues, obstetrical and gynecological issues, and traumatic injuries, such as closed-head injury, broken bones, and blunt force trauma. Trafficked persons may also seek care for medical and mental health conditions unrelated to their trafficking experiences (Baldwin et al. 2011; Kiss et al. 2015; Lederer and Wetzel 2014; Nguyen et al. 2018; Ottisova et al. 2016). Numerous barriers exist, however, to the identification of trafficked patients, as reflected in Jorge's story. In this chapter, we focus on barriers that can make identification of trafficked persons in health care settings challenging.

Studies reflect that although most trafficked individuals see an HCP at some point while trafficked, as did Jorge, they are frequently not identified or misdiagnosed (Baldwin et al. 2011; Chisolm-Straker et al. 2016; Lederer and Wetzel 2014). Missed opportunities for identification of trafficked patients are exemplified by the finding of Lederer and Wetzel (2014) that in a sample of 100 U.S.-born sex-trafficked adult and adolescent females, only 19.5% felt that although their doctor may have realized they were involved in commercial sex, no clinician inquired further. A study of 41 U.S. minors trafficked for sex who were ultimately referred to a hospital's child protection clinic found, when records were examined retrospectively, that 81% had been seen by a medical provider in the year prior (Goldberg et al. 2017).

Many variables contribute to the lack of identification and misdiagnosis. Oftentimes, as with Jorge, impediments to identification are multifactorial, a combination of victim, provider, and health system issues that interact synergistically and result in a lack of trafficked person self-disclosure and/or provider identification of the patient's exploited status (Chisolm-Straker et al. 2012; Macias-Konstantopoulos et al. 2013; Recknor et al. 2018). Failure to identify a patient as trafficked, and to understand his or her circumstances, can lead to noncompliance with the prescribed treatment plan. This in turn can lead to unimproved or worsened health outcomes, and missed opportunities for referrals to agencies that can assist with nonmedical needs, and in leaving the trafficker, if the patient chooses (Baldwin et al. 2015; Gordon et al. 2018a; Macias-Konstantopoulos 2017; Ravi et al. 2017a; Recknor et al. 2018). In this chapter, we discuss victim, provider, and health care system barriers that can inhibit recognition and the provision of care to trafficked persons. Enhanced understanding of these factors should facilitate improved identification of trafficked individuals in health care settings.

SYSTEM BARRIERS

Numerous system factors are considered barriers to identification. These factors may include the lack of organizational policies, procedures, and validated screening tools, as well as the absence of specialized practitioners and constraints on time and privacy (Table 4–1). Any of these elements alone or compounded by additional system factors and/or victim and provider barriers can inhibit victim disclosure and clinician identification.

Lack of Organizational Policies, Procedures, and Validated Screening Tools

A lack of institutional guidance on how to identify and respond to suspected trafficked persons and to access knowledge about what community resources are available for referral are obstacles to these patients receiving help within the health care system (Chisolm-Straker et al. 2012; Machtinger et al. 2019; Macias-Konstantopoulos et al. 2013; Recknor et al. 2018; Stoklosa et al. 2015). Although a growing number of health care entities realize that trafficking can

TABLE 4-1. System, provider, and victim barriers to identification

SYSTEM	PROVIDER	VICTIM
Lack of organizational policies, procedures, and validated screening tools	Lack awareness and knowledge of human trafficking	Language and cultural barriers
Limited empirical knowledge of best health care provider response to trafficked persons	Misconceptions, stereotypes, and unconscious bias	Coercive tactics of trafficker
	Discomfort with disquieting information and/or possibility of secondary traumatic stress	Fears of trafficker retaliation, arrest, and deportation
Absence of trauma-informed and human trafficking–specialized practitioners		Mistrust
		Shame and stigma
	Complex clinical presentations	Trauma bonding with the trafficker
Constraints on time and privacy		Lack of awareness of self as victim
Multiple competing priorities		Lack of knowledge of viable alternatives

occur within their patient populations, the extent to which protocols and referral networks have been established has not been documented (Stoklosa et al. 2017a, 2017c).

The lack of adequate institutional guidance on the identification of, response to, and referral of patients suspected to be trafficked can lead to provider hesitancy to assess for trafficking (Beck et al. 2015; Chisolm-Straker et al. 2012; Macias-Konstantopoulos et al. 2013; Recknor et al. 2018; Stoklosa et al. 2015). Clinicians subscribe to the bioethical principle of nonmaleficence, or "first do no harm" (Rollins et al. 2017). Believing that their actions might bring about more harm than good, providers may decide to take no action. This could include situations, for example, in which the HCP feels unable to guarantee a patient's safety, the patient is left with inadequate follow-up assistance, and/or intervention precipitates deportation or arrest (Atkinson et al. 2016; Macias-Konstantopoulos 2016; Macias-Konstantopoulos et al. 2015; Recknor et al. 2018; Rollins et al. 2017). Trafficked patients, sensing that there are inadequate community resources to help them and/or no safe place for them to go, may choose not to say anything, perceiving the situation to be hopeless (Recknor et al. 2018).

Compounding the lack of institutional policies and procedures is a dearth in human trafficking screening tools validated for both health care and mental health settings. Although HCPs may ask screening questions, if they are not using questions validated for their particular clinical settings and patient populations, misidentification may occur (Bespalova et al. 2016; C.L. Miller et al. 2016). At the time of this writing, only one validated screening tool is available, and that is specifically for 13- to 17-year-old sex-trafficked English speakers presenting in pediatric emergency departments (EDs) (see Chapter 3). There are no validated screening tools yet for adult patients in EDs (Chisolm-Straker 2018; Greenbaum et al. 2018). Neither are there tools for individuals trafficked for labor or who have chronic mental illness, who have an intellectual disability, or who are pregnant.

It is important to note that the approach of educating and providing resources, rather than simply screening, has proven efficacy for responding to domestic violence but is yet unstudied in human trafficking. These well-established health care approaches to domestic violence hold lessons for responding to trafficked persons and need further study in the human trafficking context (E. Miller et al. 2015, 2016).

Absence of Trauma-Informed, Human Trafficking–Specialized Practitioners

Health care settings vary as to availability of trauma-informed, human trafficking–specialized practitioners, such as social workers, forensic nurses, psychiatrists, psychiatric nurses, and mental health practitioners, to interview and intercede with patients when trafficking is suspected (Gordon et al. 2018b; Scannell et al. 2018). In these situations, personnel with less trauma-informed care and human trafficking expertise may be called on to work with these patients. This may lessen the likelihood of patient revelation (Lewis-O'Connor and Alpert 2017; Scannell et al. 2018).

Constraints on Time and Privacy

Health care settings are often fast paced and impersonal and do not always provide privacy. In addition, HCPs are subject to time constraints and the need to simultaneously balance multiple priorities. In many health care settings, physical space is a limited commodity. Under constraints of time, space, and competing interests, clinicians may at times speak with patients in nonprivate places such as curtained ED bays or hallways (Stoklosa et al. 2018). Combining these limitations with a lack of readily available certified interpreters, HCPs may use patient companions as interpreters when encountering a patient who speaks a different language; this is problematic if the companion is the trafficker or trafficker's accomplice. Under any or all of the enumerated circumstances, trafficked persons may not feel safe or comfortable enough to disclose their situation, and clinicians might miss trafficking indicators and/or be challenged in establishing the rapport and trust the patient needs to reveal his or her circumstances (Ahn et al. 2013; Baldwin et al. 2011; Gibbons and Stoklosa 2016; Greenbaum 2017; C.L. Miller et al. 2016; Stoklosa et al. 2018).

PROVIDER BARRIERS

Provider barriers include clinician lack of awareness and knowledge of trafficking, misconceptions and stereotypes, discomfort with disquieting information and/or the secondary traumatic stress it can engender, and the complexity of patient presentations (Table 4–1). These specific barriers can hinder HCP recognition of human trafficking. Provider factors alone, or in combination with system and/or victim barriers, can impede a trafficked patient's willingness to disclose their circumstances.

Lack of Health Care Provider Awareness and Knowledge

Provider lack of awareness of and knowledge about trafficking is frequently cited as an identification impediment (Baldwin et al. 2011; Macias-Konstantopoulos 2016). To identify trafficking, HCPs must first recognize it. Studies in multiple countries, however, document an overall lack of awareness and knowledge among clinicians (Arulrajah and Steele 2018; Chisolm-Straker et al. 2012; Long and Dowdell 2018; Recknor et al. 2018; Viergever et al. 2015). For instance, in a 2015 U.K. survey of 782 National Health Service professionals working in locales with five or more police-identified trafficking victims, only 13% of surveyed health professionals reported prior contact with known or suspected trafficked individuals, 87% reported a knowledge deficit in potential screening questions, and 78% recounted insufficient training to effectuate an appropriate response (Ross et al. 2015). Studies also reflect awareness of and knowledge about labor trafficking to be markedly limited. A 2018 qualitative study of 44 U.S. HCPs reported that although most were aware of the existence of labor trafficking, few had seen it or understood how to discern patients with everyday job injuries from patients whose injuries occurred in a situation of labor trafficking (Recknor et al. 2018).

Misconceptions and Stereotypes

HCPs can also have misconceptions and/or stereotypes about what trafficked persons look like or what constitutes trafficking, and this can hinder recognition (Barnes and Gibbs 2017; Kerr 2016; Long and Dowdell 2018; Recknor et al. 2018). Common misconceptions might include beliefs that most trafficking is for sex, in which case labor trafficking does not enter the provider's differential diagnosis (Recknor et al. 2018); that human trafficking and smuggling are the same (Barnes and Gibbs 2017); and that victims are young white females (Albright and D'Adamo 2017) or foreign-born women trafficked for sex (Long and Dowdell 2018). Clinicians adhering to these erroneous beliefs and others may not recognize trafficked persons who do not fit their narratives, potentially leaving these persons unidentified. In the case of sex trafficking, if providers only perceive females as potential victims of this crime, young males, the LGBTQ community, and other high-risk groups may not be screened for trafficking, thus leaving them unassisted (Friedman 2013; Greenbaum 2017; Rafferty 2016).

The judgmental and discriminatory attitudes associated with stereotypes can also impede identification (Bespalova et al. 2016; Coverdale et al. 2016; Long and Dowdell 2018; Macias-Konstantopoulos et al. 2013, 2015; Rajaram and Tidball 2018; Recknor et al. 2018). One such attitude is a bias against those engaged in commercial sex, or "prostitutes."[1] Members of society and HCPs alike can have difficulty understanding the difference between commercial sex and sex trafficking. As a result, trafficked individuals can experience the discriminatory attitudes that are bestowed on "prostitutes." Even with the realization that an individual has been trafficked for sex, he or she might still be stigmatized and blamed be-

---

[1]The word "prostitutes" is placed in quotation marks. Although some in health care continue to use this word, it is a legal term that refers to crime perpetration and may be perceived as conveying judgment. Both trafficked patients and those voluntarily engaged in commercial sex may perceive this bias and decide not to disclose information pertinent to their care.

cause of difficulty in understanding why an individual cannot walk away from his or her circumstances (Rajaram and Tidball 2018; Recknor et al. 2018). Furthermore, when a trafficked patient has a history of mental illness and/or substance use disorder, the clinician may doubt the veracity of that patient's story because of an unconscious bias of the clinician toward those who have histories of mental illness and/or substance use disorder (Stoklosa et al. 2017b). Clinicians displaying judgmental attitudes, or the trafficked person's anticipation of them, can elicit shame in individuals trafficked for both labor and sex, who may then choose not to disclose their situation.

Provider Discomfort

Provider discomfort with the potentially disquieting information he or she might hear when assessing for trafficking can lead to a hesitancy to ask patients questions about their experiences (Nguyen et al. 2017). HCPs wishing to deflect their own perplexity may avoid asking about what they do not wish to hear (Coverdale et al. 2016; Salami et al. 2018). Patients perceiving provider discomfort with distressing information may decide not to disclose their experiences (Baldwin et al. 2011; Lederer and Wetzel 2014).

Provider unease with certain patient behaviors can thwart identification of trafficked persons. Guardedness, streetwise demeanors, aggression and belligerence, refutation of victimhood and a need for assistance, and protectiveness and/or affection toward a seeming exploiter can be manifestations of deeper issues. These can include fear, psychological stress, dependence on and/or traumatic bonding with the abuser, and denial. HCPs not looking beneath the surface may miss opportunities to identify trafficked patients (Barnert et al. 2017; Becker and Bechtel 2015; Greenbaum 2017; Macias-Konstantopoulos et al. 2013; C.L. Miller et al. 2016). Especially in the case of sex-trafficked minors, which simply requires the confirmation of commercial sexual activity (for minors, force, fraud, or coercion need not be present according to many trafficking laws), providers' lack of clarity about what constitutes human trafficking of minors, coupled with incongruent patient behavior, can lead to underidentification (Macias-Konstantopoulos and Bar-Halpern 2016).

Complex Presentation

Clinical encounters with trafficked patients can be quite complex, making a differential diagnosis challenging and not always accurate (Gibbons and Stoklosa 2016; Macias-Konstantopoulos and Bar-

Halpern 2016; Nguyen et al. 2017; Scannell et al. 2018; Stoklosa et al. 2017a). Contrary to popular belief, trafficked individuals do not always present with symptoms suggestive of the type of abuse they have experienced (Chisolm-Straker 2018; Nguyen et al. 2018). For instance, in sex trafficking, although recurrent sexually transmitted infections could be the chief complaint, manifesting symptoms might also be vague and nonspecific; suggestive of sexual assault, domestic violence, or commercial sex; or indicative of substance use disorders, mental health issues, suicidality, and/or other psychiatric disorders (Chisolm-Straker 2018; Coverdale et al. 2016; Egyud et al. 2017; Gibbons and Stoklosa 2016; Nguyen et al. 2017; Patel et al. 2010; Ravi et al. 2017b; Stoklosa et al. 2017a).

VICTIM BARRIERS

Extant literature reflects that trafficked persons typically do not self-identify their exploitation to HCPs (Baldwin et al. 2011; Lederer and Wetzel 2014; Macias-Konstantopoulos et al. 2013; C.L. Miller et al. 2016). This compounds health care system and provider barriers and further diminishes possibilities for identification and assistance in health care settings (Macias-Konstantopoulos et al. 2013). The lack of self-disclosure can be attributed to numerous reasons. Many of these reasons are not germane to interactions with HCPs and are typical of trafficked persons' encounters with others outside of the trafficking situation (Rafferty 2016). Reasons can include language and cultural barriers; trafficker coercive tactics; fears of trafficker re-taliation, arrest, or deportation; and feelings of mistrust and shame/stigma and of being judged or ridiculed. Some trafficked persons may not perceive themselves to be victims, possibly because of trauma bonding or the belief that the situation is their choice. Others, facing economic challenges, may see no viable alternative to their current circumstances, so they remain entrenched (Table 4–1) (Baldwin et al. 2011; Lederer and Wetzel 2014; Macias-Konstantopoulos et al. 2013; C.L. Miller et al. 2016; Rafferty 2016).

SPECIAL POPULATIONS

Children and Youth

Issues pertinent to children and youth can make their identification as trafficked persons particularly challenging. For instance, in the

United States, depending on their developmental age, minors are largely thought to lack the maturity, executive functioning, and the life experiences needed to discern dangers, assess options, and restrain from immediate gratification long enough to recognize exploitation (Greenbaum 2017). Although U.S. federal anti-trafficking legislation stipulates that individuals ages 18 years or younger cannot provide consent for commercial sex, how this is interpreted from state to state varies. In some states, minors are diverted to the juvenile justice system and in others to child welfare services (Barnert et al. 2017). Regardless of the level of agency that minors perceive they have exercised in their lifestyle choices, U.S. HCPs are mandated reporters and must adhere to the laws of their state. Minors who are aware of this, and not wishing to become enmeshed in either the juvenile justice and/or child welfare system or returned to these systems, may be careful not to disclose information that would alert the HCP of a need to contact authorities (Beck et al. 2015). And just as adults may seek health care with a controlling companion who is the trafficker or an accomplice, minors might come to medical/mental health care settings with the trafficker who represents himself or herself as a parent, guardian, or family friend (Greenbaum 2017). It is also a possibility that a family member can be the trafficker (Sprang and Cole 2018). In either case, the child is unlikely to disclose information.

Psychiatric Patients

Patients with poorly managed psychiatric conditions, including complex trauma, also pose unique challenges to identification (Gibbons and Stoklosa 2016; Nguyen et al. 2017, 2018; Stoklosa et al. 2017a). If a patient presents to an ED or inpatient psychiatry unit in a decompensated state and unable to report an accurate history, emergent literature recommends rescreening for trafficking after stabilization. Also recommended is the need for constant surveillance for trafficking among psychiatric patients, particularly because many of the risk factors for exploitation are the same for those with major mental disorders (Coverdale et al. 2016; Nguyen et al. 2017, 2018).

CONCLUSION

Because of the diverse and complex nature of human trafficking, there are a plethora of system-, provider-, and victim-associated barriers to the identification and care of trafficked persons. Recognition of barriers to identification of trafficked persons in health and mental health care settings provides opportunities for HCPs and organizations to proactively address actual and potential barriers to identifying human trafficking through provider education on human trafficking, training in trauma-informed care, and implementation of organizational policies and procedures. When HCPs and organizations address barriers to recognition of trafficked persons by increasing HCP education, addressing system issues, implementing organizational policies and procedures, and increasing system and provider awareness of potential victim barriers, more trafficked persons will be identified and cared for. Increasing victim identification can mitigate adverse mental and physical health outcomes for victims acutely and longitudinally. Importantly, adopting measures to break through the barriers inhibiting recognition will increase the HCP's confidence and competence in providing care for this population.

Pearls and Pointers

- Health professionals should be aware of the role that system barriers may play in trafficking and seek creative solutions. For example, ensure patient privacy for conversations about abuse.
- Health professionals should be aware of trafficked person–related barriers to disclosure.
- Universal application of trauma-informed, culturally competent approaches may mitigate system, provider, and patient barriers to human trafficking identification.
- Health professionals should acknowledge their own unconscious biases related to patient populations vulnerable to trafficking.

REFERENCES

Ahn R, Alpert EJ, Purcell G, et al: Human trafficking: review of educational resources for health professionals. Am J Prev Med 44(3):283–289, 2013 23415126

Albright E, D'Adamo K: The media and human trafficking: a discussion and critique of the dominant narrative, in Human Trafficking is a Public Health Issue: A Paradigm Expansion in the United States. Edited by Chisolm-Straker M, Stoklosa H. Cham, Switzerland, Springer, 2017, pp 363–378

Arulrajah P, Steele S: UK medical education on human trafficking: assessing uptake of the opportunity to shape awareness, safeguarding and referral in the curriculum. BMC Med Educ 18(1):137, 2018 29895263

Atkinson HG, Curnin KJ, Hanson NC: U.S. state laws addressing human trafficking: education of and mandatory reporting by health care providers and other professionals. Journal of Human Trafficking 2(2):111–138, 2016

Baldwin SB, Eisenman DP, Sayles JN, et al: Identification of human trafficking victims in health care settings. Health Hum Rights 13(1):E36–E49, 2011 22772961

Baldwin SB, Fehrenbacher AE, Eisenman DP: Psychological coercion in human trafficking: an application of Biderman's framework. Qual Health Res 25(9):1171–1181, 2015 25371382

Barnert E, Iqbal Z, Bruce J, et al: Commercial sexual exploitation and sex trafficking of children and adolescents: a narrative review. Acad Pediatr 17(8):825–829, 2017 28797913

Barnes WJ, Gibbs HA: Sex trafficked and missed, in Human Trafficking is a Public Health Issue: A Paradigm Expansion in the United States. Edited by Chisolm-Straker M, Stoklosa H. Cham, Switzerland, Springer, 2017, pp 15–27

Beck ME, Lineer MM, Melzer-Lange M, et al: Medical providers' understanding of sex trafficking and their experience with at-risk patients. Pediatrics 135(4):e895–e902, 2015 25780076

Becker HJ, Bechtel K: Recognizing victims of human trafficking in the pediatric emergency department. Pediatr Emerg Care 31(2):144–147, quiz 148–150, 2015 25651385

Bespalova N, Morgan J, Coverdale J: A pathway to freedom: an evaluation of screening tools for the identification of trafficking victims. Acad Psychiatry 40(1):124–128, 2016 25398267

Chisolm-Straker M: Measured steps: evidence-based anti-trafficking efforts in the ED. Acad Emerg Med 25(11):1302–1305, 2018 30112784

Chisolm-Straker M, Richardson LD, Cossio T: Combating slavery in the 21st century: the role of emergency medicine. J Health Care Poor Underserved 23(3):980–987, 2012 24212151

Chisolm-Straker M, Baldwin S, Gaïgbé-Togbé B, et al: Health care and human trafficking: we are seeing the unseen. J Health Care Poor Underserved 27(3):1220–1233, 2016 27524764

Coverdale J, Beresin EV, Louie AK, et al: Human trafficking and psychiatric education: a call to action. Acad Psychiatry 40(1):119–123, 2016 26670788

Egyud A, Stephens K, Swanson-Bierman B, et al: Implementation of human trafficking education and treatment algorithm in the emergency department. J Emerg Nurs 43(6):526–531, 2017 28427727

Friedman SA: And boys too: an ECPAT discussion paper about the lack of recognition of the commercial sexual exploitation of boys in the United States. 2013. Available at: https://static1.squarespace.com/static/594970e91b631b3571be12e2/t/5977b2dacd0f688b2b89e6f0/1501016795183/ECPAT-USA_AndBoysToo.pdf. Accessed October 29, 2019.

Gibbons P, Stoklosa H: Identification and treatment of human trafficking victims in the emergency department: a case report. J Emerg Med 50(5):715–719, 2016 26896287

Goldberg AP, Moore JL, Houck C, et al: Domestic minor sex trafficking patients: a retrospective analysis of medical presentation. J Pediatr Adolesc Gynecol 30(1):109–115, 2017 27575407

Gordon M, Fang S, Coverdale J, et al: Failure to identify a human trafficking victim. Am J Psychiatry 175(5):408–409, 2018a 29712468

Gordon M, Salami T, Coverdale J, et al: Psychiatry's role in the management of human trafficking victims: an integrated care approach. J Psychiatr Pract 24(2):79–86, 2018b 29509177

Greenbaum VJ: Child sex trafficking in the United States: Challenges for the healthcare provider. PLoS Med 14(11):e1002439, 2017 29166405

Greenbaum VJ, Dodd M, McCracken C: A short screening tool to identify victims of child sex trafficking in the health care setting. Pediatr Emerg Care 34(1):33–37, 2018 26599463

Kerr P: Treating trauma in the context of human trafficking: intersections of psychological, social, and cultural factors, in International Perspectives on Traumatic Stress. Edited by Ghafoori B, Caspi Y, Smith SF. New York, Nova Science Publishers, 2016, pp 199–221

Kiss L, Pocock NS, Naisanguansri V, et al: Health of men, women, and children in post-trafficking services in Cambodia, Thailand, and Vietnam: an observational cross-sectional study. Lancet Glob Health 3(3):e154–e161, 2015 25701993

Lederer LJ, Wetzel C: The health consequences of sex trafficking and their implications for identifying victims in health care facilities. Annals of Health Law 23(1):61–91, 2014

Lewis-O'Connor A, Alpert EJ: Caring for survivors using a trauma-informed care framework, in Human Trafficking is a Public Health Issue: A Paradigm Expansion in the United States. Edited by Chisolm-Straker M, Stoklosa H. Cham, Switzerland, Springer, 2017, pp 309–323

Long E, Dowdell EB: Nurses' perceptions of victims of human trafficking in an urban emergency department: a qualitative study. J Emerg Nurs 44(4):375–383, 2018 29254652

Machtinger E, Davis K, Kimberg L, et al: From treatment to healing: inquiry and response to recent and past trauma in adult health care. Women's Health Issues 29(2):97–102, 2019 30606467

Macias-Konstantopoulos WL: Human trafficking: the role of medicine in interrupting the cycle of abuse and violence. Ann Intern Med 165(8):582–588, 2016 27537695

Macias-Konstantopoulos WL: Caring for the trafficked patient: ethical challenges and recommendations for health care professionals. AMA J Ethics 19(1):80–90, 2017 28107159

Macias-Konstantopoulos WL, Bar-Halpern M: Commercially sexually exploited and trafficked minors: our hidden and forgotten children, in Stigma and Prejudice: Touchstones in Understanding Diversity in Healthcare. Edited by Parekh R, Childs EW. Cham, Switzerland, Springer, 2016, pp 183–202

Macias-Konstantopoulos WL, Ahn R, Alpert EJ, et al: An international comparative public health analysis of sex trafficking of women and girls in eight cities: achieving a more effective health sector response. J Urban Health 90(6):1194–1204, 2013 24151086

Macias-Konstantopoulos WL, Munroe D, Purcell G, et al: The commercial sexual exploitation and sex trafficking of minors in the Boston metropolitan area: Experiences and challenges faced by front-line providers and other stakeholders. Journal of Applied Research on Children 6(1):4, 2015

Miller CL, Duke G, Northam S: Child sex-trafficking recognition, intervention, and referral: an educational framework to the development of health care provider education programs. Journal of Human Trafficking 2(3):177–200, 2016

Miller E, Goldstein S, McCauley HL, et al: A school health center intervention for abusive adolescent relationships: a cluster RCT. Pediatrics 135(1):76–85, 2015 25535265

Miller E, Tancredi DJ, Decker MR, et al: A family planning clinic-based intervention to address reproductive coercion: a cluster randomized controlled trial. Contraception 94(1):58–67, 2016 26892333

Nguyen PT, Coverdale JH, Gordon MR: Identifying, treating, and advocating for human trafficking victims: a key role for psychiatric inpatient units. Gen Hosp Psychiatry 46:41–43, 2017 28622814

Nguyen PT, Lamkin J, Coverdale JH, et al: Identifying human trafficking victims on a psychiatry inpatient service: A case series. Psychiatr Q 89(2):341–348, 2018 28971296

Ottisova L, Hemmings S, Howard LM, et al: Prevalence and risk of violence and the mental, physical and sexual health problems associated with human trafficking: an updated systematic review. Epidemiol Psychiatr Sci 25(4):317–341, 2016 27066701

Patel RB, Ahn R, Burke TF: Human trafficking in the emergency department. West J Emerg Med 11(5):402–404, 2010 21293753

Powell C, Asbill M, Louis E, et al: Identifying gaps in human trafficking mental health service provision. Journal of Human Trafficking 4(3):256–269, 2018

Rafferty Y: Challenges to the rapid identification of children who have been trafficked for commercial sexual exploitation. Child Abuse Negl 52:158–168, 2016 26718261

Rajaram SS, Tidball S: Survivors' voices—complex needs of sex trafficking survivors in the Midwest. Behav Med 44(3):189–198, 2018 29095121

Ravi A, Pfeiffer MR, Rosner Z, et al: Identifying health experiences of domestically sex-trafficked women in the USA: a qualitative study in Rikers Island Jail. J Urban Health 94(3):408–416, 2017a 28116589

Ravi A, Pfeiffer MR, Rosner Z, et al: Trafficking and trauma: insight and advice for the healthcare system from sex-trafficked women incarcerated on Rikers Island. Med Care 55(12):1017–1022, 2017b 28945674

Recknor FH, Gemeinhardt G, Selwyn BJ: Health-care provider challenges to the identification of human trafficking in health-care settings: a qualitative study. Journal of Human Trafficking 4(3):213–230, 2018

Rollins R, Gribble A, Barrett SE, et al: Who is in your waiting room? Health care professionals as culturally responsive and trauma-informed first responders to human trafficking. AMA J Ethics 19(1):63–71, 2017 28107157

Ross C, Dimitrova S, Howard LM, et al: Human trafficking and health: a cross-sectional survey of NHS professionals' contact with victims of human trafficking. BMJ Open 5(8):e008682, 2015 26293659

Salami T, Gordon M, Coverdale J, et al: What therapies are favored in the treatment of the psychological sequelae of trauma in human trafficking victims? J Psychiatr Pract 24(2):87–96, 2018 29509178

Scannell M, MacDonald AE, Berger A, et al: Human trafficking: how nurses can make a difference. J Forensic Nurs 14(2):117–121, 2018 29781972

Sprang G, Cole J: Familial sex trafficking of minors: trafficking conditions, clinical presentation, and system involvement. Journal of Family Violence 33(3):185–195, 2018

Stoklosa H, Grace AM, Littenberg N: Medical education on human trafficking. AMA J Ethics 17(10):914–921, 2015 26496054

Stoklosa H, Dawson MB, Williams-Oni F, et al: A review of US health care institution protocols for the identification and treatment of victims of human trafficking. Journal of Human Trafficking 3(2):116–124, 2017a

Stoklosa H, MacGibbon M, Stoklosa J: Human trafficking, mental illness, and addiction: avoiding diagnostic overshadowing. AMA J Ethics 19(1):23–34, 2017b 28107153

Stoklosa H, Showalter H, Melnick A, et al: Health care providers' experience with a protocol for the identification, treatment, and referral of human trafficking victims. Journal of Human Trafficking 3(3):182–192, 2017c

Stoklosa H, Scannell M, Ma Z, et al: Do EPs change their clinical behaviour in the hallway or when a companion is present? A cross-sectional survey. Emerg Med J 35(7):406–411, 2018 29431142

Viergever RF, West H, Borland R, et al: Health care providers and human trafficking: what do they know, what do they need to know? Findings from the Middle East, the Caribbean, and Central America. Front Public Health 3:6, 2015 25688343

Emergency Department Management of Trafficked Persons

Zheng Ben Ma, M.D.

Hanni Stoklosa, M.D., M.P.H.

> One compassionate gaze or one affectionate handshake can substitute for years of friendship when a person is in agony. Not only does love last forever, it needs only a second to be born.
>
> —*Henri Nouwen,* The Wounded Healer *(1972)*

An 18-year-old transgender male presents to the emergency department (ED) with a fentanyl overdose. He is unconscious, and the emergency providers begin resuscitating him, administering bag-mask ventilation and medicating with naloxone. Trauma shears are used to remove his clothing, and multiple bags of cocaine are found tucked in his pockets and in his boxer shorts. After treatment with naloxone, he regains consciousness, immediately looks for his backpack, and becomes agitated, shouting, "Who took my backpack?" and "Where are my pants?" A review of his chart shows he has a history of bipolar disorder, prior child welfare involvement, prior incarcerations, and polysubstance use. He was later discharged against medical advice.

He did not disclose to his health care providers that he has been living on the street and is having trouble paying for his hormone treatments. To pay for his hormone treatments, he started selling drugs for an older man. Initially, things were fine, and then the older man started telling him he had to sell more and more, and if he did not meet the quotas, he was threatened with beatings. Sometimes, he was punished with gang rape.

ENCOUNTERING AND IDENTIFYING TRAFFICKED PERSONS IN THE EMERGENCY DEPARTMENT

Emergency providers (physicians, mental health workers, nurses, and other essential staff) may be the first caring professionals to encounter a trafficked person. The nature of emergency medicine allows for interaction with patients from all different demographics, socioeconomic statuses, and racial and ethnic groups, as well as with many disease varieties and severities. Within a U.S. trafficking survivor cohort, the most commonly visited site for medical care was the hospital ED, where 63% of the cohort reported receiving treatment (Lederer and Wetzel 2014). It is crucial that the emergency provider understand that a trafficked person can present to the ED from any demographic group and with any type of complaint; the provider must take care to avoid functioning with a preconceived, narrow perception of which patient may have experienced human trafficking.

The definition of a human trafficking victim, according to the Trafficking Victims Protection Act of 2000 (P.L. 106-386), does not necessitate physical movement across any borders. According to a special report from the U.S. Department of Justice, 83% of victims of confirmed sex-trafficking incidents were identified as U.S. citizens (Banks and Kyckelhahn 2011). Health care providers in the ED should therefore maintain an index of suspicion even for patients who reside within their local communities. Additionally, according to federal law, any case of a minor less than the age of 18 years who is involved in commercial sex is considered trafficked by sexual exploitation (P.L. 106-386). Therefore, any minor who presents with issues that raise concerns related to sexual exploitation should trigger a provider's suspicions.

The topic of human trafficking is gaining increased attention in both the popular media and within health care disciplines. However, the dominant perception of a trafficked person is that of a young female involved in the sex trade (Albright and D'Adamo 2017). This perception stands in contrast to the International Labour Organization's estimates that labor trafficking comprises 68% of individuals who have been trafficked worldwide (International Labour Organization 2012). Within the United States, "trafficking occurs in both legal and illicit industries, including in commercial sex, hospitality, traveling sales crews, agriculture, janitorial services, construction, restaurants, care for persons with disabilities, salon services, massage parlors, fairs and carnivals, peddling and begging, drug smuggling and distribution, and child care and domestic work" (U.S. Department of State 2018, p. 448). Although globally women and girls account for an estimated 71% of modern slavery victims, providers should not be falsely reassured if their patient is male or if their patient is involved in a legal or "legitimate" industry (United Nations Office on Drugs and Crimes 2016). Nevertheless, certain populations are at increased risk for exploitation as noted in Table 5–1.

For various reasons, trafficked persons will rarely self-identify or report their abuse while seeking medical care. Barriers to self-identification, for example, may include feelings of shame or guilt, fear of retaliation, fear of arrest, and lack of understanding of the U.S. health care system (National Human Trafficking Resource Center 2016b). In fact, trafficked persons may have been coached by their traffickers on responses to anticipated questions from health care providers to divert suspicion by portraying a seemingly innocuous story. Understanding what to look for in recognizing a patient as a potential trafficked person is a crucial first step to identifying a trafficked person. Several indicators may help emergency providers become alerted to the possibility of their patient's potential trafficking victim status as outlined in Table 5–1.

ADDRESSING HEALTH EFFECTS OF HUMAN TRAFFICKING

The emergency provider's priority for potential victims of trafficking, as with all patients, is to address the acute and potentially life-threatening illnesses and injuries of their patients. Whether it is septic complications of a sexually transmitted infection or particularly severe traumatic injuries, stabilizing life- or limb-threatening injuries is the expertise of emergency medicine practitioners, and high-quality medical care of a potential trafficking victim should be the first focus of attention.

Nevertheless, most trafficked persons who present as patients to the ED will likely not be in a critical or unstable state and may present with any number of chief complaints within a wide range of serious health problems related to their physical, mental, and sexually abusive experiences (Chisolm-Straker et al. 2016; Oram et al. 2012). Table 5–2 highlights the spectrum of possible health effects from trafficking. Trafficked persons may suffer varying degrees of health consequences, depending on their living and working conditions. Table 5–2 should not be considered exhaustive because each individual case varies by form of abuse, and many trafficked persons may not have access to care for their various medical needs. Human trafficking often exists with concurrent substance use, violence, and psycho-

TABLE 5–1. Indicators of a potential trafficked person

GENERAL TRAFFICKING	LABOR TRAFFICKING	SEX TRAFFICKING
Scripted or inconsistent history	Has been abused at work or threatened with harm by employer or supervisor	Under age 18 and involved in commercial sex
Unwilling or hesitant to answer questions about the injury/illness	Not allowed to take adequate breaks or to have adequate access to food or water while at work	Has tattoos or other forms of branding, including "Daddy," "Property of...," "For sale," etc.
Accompanied by individual who does not allow patient to speak for themselves, does not allow them to have privacy, or interprets for them	Not provided with adequate personal protective equipment for hazardous work	Reports unusually high numbers of sexual partners
Evidence of controlling or dominating relationships (excessive concerns about pleasing a family member, partner, or employer)	Was recruited for different work than he/she is currently doing	Does not have appropriate clothing for weather or venue
Demonstrates fearful or nervous behavior or avoids eye contact	Required to live in housing provided by employer	Uses language common in commercial sex
Resistant to assistance or demonstrates hostile behavior	Has debt to owner or recruiter with significant barriers to pay off	
Unable to provide own address		
Not aware of own location, current date, or time		
Not in possession of own identification documents		
Not in control of own money		
Not being paid or wages withheld		

Source.   Adapted from National Human Trafficking Resource Center 2016a.

logical problems in the lives of patients. It is therefore important that emergency providers recognize that their patients' primary substance-related or mental health–related complaint, which brought them to the ED to seek care, may be secondary or concurrent to their active or prior exploitation from trafficking (Stoklosa et al. 2017). As a result of fear, psychological manipulation, and abuse suffered, trafficked persons will experience a similarly broad spectrum of mental health consequences. These may include feelings of intense stigma, shame, anxiety, and hopelessness, in addition to pathological fear, panic attacks, sleep disturbances, dissociative disorders, posttraumatic stress disorder, and suicidal ideation and attempts (Alpert et al. 2014; Kastrup 2013; Kiss et al. 2015; Tsutsumi et al. 2008; Zimmerman et al. 2006).

HISTORY AND PHYSICAL EXAM

Potential trafficked persons will likely not self-identify to medical providers about their abusive situations. Their harsh experiences, by the time they reach the ED, may well have eroded their trust of those perceived to be in positions of authority. Trafficked persons may also face threats to their family or loved ones, including their children. Therefore, their disclosure of abuse may lead to further harm or danger for others, making trafficked persons even more reluctant to reach out for help (Baldwin et al. 2015). The primary goal for the emergency provider is therefore not necessarily to obtain disclosure or even rescue the trafficked persons; rather, the medical provider should "work to establish the ED as a haven from trauma or exploitation and to offer available resources if possible" (Shandro et al. 2016, p. 504).

The first goal of the medical provider is to establish a trusting and caring relationship with the patient who is a potential trafficked person. Emergency providers may not have the luxury of developing this therapeutic alliance over time, but establishing rapport by using trauma-informed care principles while respecting and protecting the patient's need of confidentiality and maintaining a nonjudgmental, genuine demeanor will go a long way toward gaining the vulnerable patient's confidence, even in the briefest of encounters in the ED.

Given the sensitive nature of these topics, strong efforts should be made to assure the patient's privacy and confidentiality. Patients should ideally be placed in care areas with private and protected space instead of hallway care areas, as is increasingly common practice in many crowded EDs (Stoklosa et al. 2018). The patient should be separated from accompanying persons who may be traffickers or en-

TABLE 5–2.   Health effects of human trafficking that may be encountered in the emergency department

PHYSICAL INJURY	REPRODUCTIVE HEALTH	DEVELOPMENTAL HEALTH	COMPREHENSIVE HEALTH
Intentional and accidental burns	Genitoanal trauma or foreign body	Delayed physical and cognitive developmental milestones	Malnutrition
Branding, tattoos, and other purposeful stigmata of "ownership"	Repeated unwanted pregnancy	Stunting, vitamin deficiencies, and other consequences of chronic poor nutrition	Dental caries
Blunt force trauma	Complications from previously or repeatedly performed abortions	Impaired social skills	Headaches
Firearm and knife wounds	Sexually transmitted infections, including HIV/AIDS	Long-term effects of inadequately treated childhood diseases	Fatigue
Strangulation injuries	Chronic complications including infertility, chronic pelvic pain, cervical cancer, liver failure		Abdominal complaints
Fractures			Chronic pain syndromes
Dental and oral cavity injuries			Substance use disorders
Traumatic brain injuries			Infectious diseases usually prevented through routine immunizations
Neuropathies			Other infectious diseases such as tuberculosis, HIV, intestinal parasites, hepatitis
Scarring and other healed injuries			
Chronic musculoskeletal pain from repeated strain or overuse			
Vision and hearing impairment from lack of protective gear			
Skin, neurological, and respiratory sequalae from exposure and inhalation injuries			
Effects of prolonged heat or cold exposures			

forcers posing as the patient's family or friends. This may be achieved naturally within the workflow of ED care during times when the patient is being examined or receiving diagnostic tests or by asking the accompanying individual to complete paperwork in another care area. (Alpert et al. 2014) If the patient's primary language is not English, official interpretive services should be used rather than the patient's accompanying "family member." Meeting the patient's immediate physical needs for food, water, blanket, and so forth, when possible, is another manner of establishing trust. Furthermore, clinicians may empower the patient to decide if they feel comfortable speaking with a male or female practitioner (National Human Trafficking Resource Center 2016b).

When the patient is in a reliably safe and private care area, the provider should engage the patient with patience and respect, sitting at eye level when asking questions, maintaining eye contact, while speaking honestly and in a nonjudgmental manner (Shandro et al. 2016). Because building trust and rapport with potential trafficked persons requires time and patience, the emergency physician or practitioner may not have the appropriate amount of time necessary to have a longer discussion with the patient. In these situations, the provider should find a another time to come back to the patient when the provider can devote the appropriate time and attention to a longer discussion with the patient, or, alternatively, the emergency providers can partner with a multidisciplinary professional, such as a social worker, mental health worker, nurse, or midlevel practitioner who can meet with the patient (National Human Trafficking Resource Center 2016a).

Emergency providers should perform a physical exam that is relevant to the patient's presenting complaint but do so in a thorough manner to avoid missing potential indicators of exploitation. Special attention should be paid to signs of malnutrition, dehydration, physical exhaustion, untreated past injuries, and multiple injuries and bruises (Baldwin and Sanders 2018; Becker and Bechtel 2015). A complete skin exam may reveal marks consistent with burns, bites, ligature wounds, bruises, traumatic alopecia, scars, unhealed wounds, or tattoos resembling branding, especially in unusual locations such as the inner thigh, underarm, breast, or back of neck. The genitourinary examination may reveal evidence of sexually transmitted infections, traumatic injuries, foreign bodies, or complications from prior unsafe abortions (Shandro et al. 2016).

Although the emergency provider should aim for thoroughness in the physical exam, this goal must be balanced with the patient-centered need to respect and empower the trafficked person's sense of control. As trafficked persons suffer loss of control and autonomy in numerous aspects of their lives, empowering their sense of control in the ED will help foster their sense of trust in medical providers as a source of support (Baldwin et al. 2015). Each part of the physical exam, particularly the invasive portions such as the skin and genitourinary exams, should only be performed after obtaining the patient's permission. Additional possible findings on physical examination are listed in Table 5–2.

MANDATED REPORTING

Physicians and other clinicians are mandated reporters who are required by law to report certain cases of suspected abuse or neglect. Each state has its own relevant laws and regulations with which the emergency provider should be familiar. The revised federal Child Abuse and Prevention Treatment Act requires that states amend their child abuse laws so that mandatory reporting of child abuse includes "victims of sex trafficking or severe forms of trafficking in persons" (Justice for Victims of Trafficking Act of 2015 [P.L. 114-22]). Whenever possible, the provider should inform the patient of mandatory reporting before hearing any reportable information to give patients and potential trafficked persons as much control over the situation as possible (Chisolm-Straker 2018). Although patients do not have any control over providers' mandatory reporting requirements, patients should be informed of the limits of confidentiality and should be aware of and exercise their own choice about whether to receive additional resources or speak with other agencies. Reporting "has the potential to bring victims and survivors to the attention of social service and law enforcement agencies but may discourage trafficked persons from seeking help, thereby limiting the ability of health care professionals to establish trust and provide needed care" (English 2017, p. 54). Reporting without the knowledge of patients will almost certainly damage the hard-earned trust of trafficked persons.

TRAUMA-INFORMED CARE

The experiences of intense physical, emotional, and sexual trauma endured by trafficked persons can have complex and profound impacts on their ability to function, patterns of behavior, and sense of self-identity. The emergency provider should provide care for trafficked persons in a trauma-informed manner to best support and empower patients while avoiding retraumatization.

The tenets of trauma-informed care include the following (Substance Abuse and Mental Health Services Administration 2014):

- *Realize* the widespread impact of trauma and understand potential paths for recovery.
- *Recognize* the signs and symptoms of trauma in patients, families, staff, and others involved.
- *Respond* by fully integrating knowledge into policies, procedures, and practices.
- *Seek* to actively resist retraumatization.

The goal of the trauma-informed approach to patient care is to create a safe and supportive environment for abused and exploited trafficked persons to obtain the supportive services they need while receiving affirmation and empowerment (Baldwin and Sanders 2018; National Human Trafficking Resource Center 2015). Additional interventions to foster this goal may include reducing the number of interviews asked of the patient, holding evaluations where the trafficked person feels safe, taking breaks as needed during the interview, and having an advocate present to support the trafficked person as they share their story.

A trafficked person may demonstrate a traumatic response during evaluation as evidenced by one or several of the following behaviors (National Human Trafficking Resource Center 2015):

- Exhibits gaps in memory, provides a disjointed timeline, gives narrative with inconsistencies or changing details
- Appears frozen, shut down, or disconnected from the moment
- Appears overwhelmed by sense of shame, guilt, or helplessness
- Exhibits difficulty concentrating, thinking rationally, following schedules, or making decisions
- Demonstrates hostile or angry tendencies
- Appears distrustful of others or overly reliant on others, shies away from others, or repeatedly pursues unhealthy relationships

Providers can help mitigate these responses by reaffirming the patient's sense of control, providing a break in the evaluation, normalizing the reaction, and consistently demonstrating a supportive and nonjudgmental attitude. Caring for traumatized trafficked persons who may externalize their frustrations can be a challenging experience for the emergency provider. Those in the provider role should not take any of the trafficked persons' reactions personally and should seek their own emotional supportive measures as needed. Educational resources exist for trauma-informed training for health care providers, and resources continue to grow in number as this issue is becoming better recognized. EDs and hospital organizations should make efforts to train their staff in all patient care roles and to provide appropriate trauma-informed trainings to ensure optimal care of potential trafficked persons.

REFERRAL FOR ADDITIONAL RESOURCES

A key resource with which every health care provider should be familiar is the National Human Trafficking Hotline at 1-888-373-7888. The National Human Trafficking Hotline is a service available 24 hours every day of the year to trafficked persons, survivors, and health care providers alike. Staff members are trained to assist in a manner compliant with the Health Insurance Portability and Accountability Act (HIPAA) and can provide callers from any background with local resources including shelter, legal services, and law enforcement referrals (Powell et al. 2018). A potential trafficked person may call this resource at any stage of their exploitation to be connected to resources.

When seeking resources, the provider and patient should consider the impact of engaging law enforcement. Many trafficked persons have had poor experiences with law enforcement officials and legitimately have a fear of arrest or deportation or of suffering abuse at the hands of authority figures in general (Restore NYC 2019; Stoklosa and Baldwin 2017; Zimmerman and Borland 2009). Nevertheless, some mandated reporting laws require the provider to report suspected human trafficking to law enforcement. Whenever possible, try to partner with the patient—and with trusted law enforcement personnel—in these decisions and allow the patient control over confidential and personal details.

Although dramatic but discrete measures, such as hiding a small piece of paper with the National Human Trafficking Hotline number in a shoe or on small trinkets have been described, the provider should carefully consider the specific situation of the trafficked person (Shandro et al. 2016). Sometimes providing such information may pose a risk to the patient's safety. A safer route would be to post available resources in private spaces such as the ED bathroom so that the patient can memorize the information instead.

CONCLUSION

Caring for the potential trafficked person is a challenging responsibility for the emergency provider (Shandro et al. 2016). All providers should be trained to recognize possible trafficked persons and to provide sensitive, trauma-informed care to help establish the ED as a safe space. The first priority for the emergency provider is to care for the patient's medical and bodily needs. Subsequent referral to trafficking-specific resources and follow-up care should be considered thoughtfully, with as much patient input and control as possible. Although the process is difficult, the stakes are incredibly high. Few interventions in the ED can have as profound an impact on patients' lives as the care provided to the trafficked person.

Pearls and Pointers

- Trafficked persons can present to the emergency department (ED) from any demographic group and with any chief complaint.
- The emergency provider's first priority is to address the health and bodily needs of the potential trafficked person.
- The goal of the ED visit is not to seek disclosure from the trafficked person but rather to establish trust and respect and offer appropriate resources.
- Emergency providers should care for potential trafficked persons in a trauma-informed manner while empowering the patient with as much control as possible.
- Emergency providers should be aware of local resources for trafficked persons and thoughtfully employ a multidisciplinary team to best care for patients' needs.

REFERENCES

Albright E, D'Adamo K: The media and human trafficking: a discussion and critique of the dominant narrative, in Human Trafficking Is a Public Health Issue. Edited by Chisolm-Straker M, Stoklosa H. Cham, Switzerland, Springer, 2017, pp 363–378

Alpert EJ, Ahn R, Albright E, et al: Human Trafficking: Guidebook on Identification, Assessment, and Response in the Health Care Setting. Waltham, MA, Massachusetts Medical Society, 2014

Baldwin S, Sanders S: Identifying + responding to human trafficking in health care settings. Essential Access Health Webinar, November 28, 2018. Available at: www.essentialaccess.org/learning-exchange/identifying-responding-human-trafficking-health-care-settings-2018. Accessed October 30, 2019.

Baldwin SB, Fehrenbacher AE, Eisenman DP: Psychological coercion in human trafficking: an application of Biderman's framework. Qual Health Res 25(9):1171–1181, 2015 25371382

Banks D, Kyckelhahn T: Characteristics of suspected human trafficking incidents, 2008–2010. Washington, DC, U.S. Department of Justice, Office of Justice Programs, Bureau of Justice Statistics, 2011

Becker HJ, Bechtel K: Recognizing victims of human trafficking in the pediatric emergency department. Pediatr Emerg Care 31(2):144–147, quiz 148–150, 2015 25651385

Chisolm-Straker M: Managing trafficking in the pediatric ED. Empire State EPIC 36(2):19–22, 2018

Chisolm-Straker M, Baldwin S, Gaïgbé-Togbé B, et al: Health care and human trafficking: we are seeing the unseen. J Health Care Poor Underserved 27(3):1220–1233, 2016 27524764

English A: Mandatory reporting of human trafficking: potential benefits and risks of harm. AMA J Ethics 19(1):54–62, 2017 28107156

International Labour Organization: ILO Global Estimate of Forced Labour 2012: Results and Methodology. Geneva, International Labour Office, Special Action Programme to Combat Forced Labour, 2012. Available at: www.ilo.org/wcmsp5/groups/public/---ed_norm/---declaration/documents/publication/wcms_182004.pdf. Accessed October 30, 2019.

Justice for Victims of Trafficking Act of 2015, Pub. L. No. 114-22 (129 STAT.227) 2015

Kastrup M: Abuse and trafficking among female migrants and refugees, in Violence Against Women and Mental Health. Edited by García-Moreno C, Riecher-Rössler A. Basel, Switzerland, Karger Publishers, 2013, pp 118–128

Kiss L, Pocock NS, Naisanguansri V, et al: Health of men, women, and children in post-trafficking services in Cambodia, Thailand, and Vietnam: an observational cross-sectional study. Lancet Glob Health 3(3):e154–e161, 2015 25701993

Lederer LJ, Wetzel CA: The health consequences of sex trafficking and their implications for identifying victims in healthcare facilities. Annals of Health Law 23(1):61–87, 2014

National Human Trafficking Resource Center: Trauma-informed human trafficking screenings. 2015. Available at: https://humantraffickinghotline.org/resources/trauma-informed-human-trafficking-screenings. Accessed October 30, 2019.

National Human Trafficking Resource Center: Identifying victims of human trafficking: what to look for in a healthcare setting. February 16, 2016a. Available at: https://traffickingresourcecenter.org/sites/default/files/What%20to%20Look%20for%20during%20a%20Medical%20Exam%20-%20FINAL%20-%202-16-16.docx.pdf. Accessed October 30, 2019.

National Human Trafficking Resource Center: Recognizing and responding to human trafficking in a healthcare context. 2012. Updated 2016b. Available at: https://humantraffickinghotline.org/sites/default/files/ Recognizing%20and %20Responding%20to%20Human%20Trafficking%20in%20a%20 Healthcare%20Context_pdf.pdf. Accessed October 30, 2019.

Nouwen H: The Wounded Healer. New York, Doubleday, 1972

Oram S, Stockl H, Busza J, et al: Prevalence and risk of violence and the physical, mental, and sexual health problems associated with human trafficking: systematic review. PLoS medicine 9(5):e1001224, 2012 22666182

Powell C, Asbill M, Brew S, et al: Human trafficking and HIPAA: what the health care professional needs to know. Journal of Human Trafficking 4(2):105–113, 2018

Restore NYC: Healthcare access for foreign-national survivors of trafficking. 2019. Available at: https://static1.squarespace.com/static/ 59d51bdb6f4ca3f65e5a8d07/t/5c38a0b9032be4443a65a961/ 1547215052741/HC+PAPER+FINAL.pdf. Accessed October 30, 2019.

Shandro J, Chisolm-Straker M, Duber HC, et al: Human trafficking: a guide to identification and approach for the emergency physician. Ann Emerg Med 68(4):501–508.e1, 2016 27130802

Stoklosa H, Baldwin SB: Health professional education on trafficking: the facts matter. Lancet 390(10103):1641–1642, 2017 28939094

Stoklosa H, Stoklosa JB, MacGibbon M: Human trafficking, mental illness, and addiction: avoiding diagnostic overshadowing. AMA J Ethics 19(1):22–34, 2017 28107156

Stoklosa H, Stoklosa JB, MacGibbon M, et al: Do EPs change their clinical behaviour in the hallway or when a companion is present? A cross-sectional survey. Emerg Med J 35(7):406–411, 2018 29431142

Substance Abuse and Mental Health Services Administration: SAMHSA's concept of trauma and guidance for a trauma-informed approach. July 2014. Available at: https://store.samhsa.gov/system/files/sma14-4884.pdf. Accessed October 30, 2019.

Trafficking Victims Protection Act of 2000, Pub. L. No. 106-386

Tsutsumi A, Izutsu T, Poudyal AK, et al: Mental health of female survivors of human trafficking in Nepal. Soc Sci Med 66(8):1841–1847, 2008 18276050

United Nations Office on Drugs and Crime: Global Report on Trafficking in Persons. Vienna, United Nations Office on Drugs and Crime, 2016. Available at: www.unodc.org/documents/data-and-analysis/glotip/ 2016_Global_Report_on_Trafficking_in_Persons.pdf. Accessed October 30, 2019.

U.S. Department of State: Trafficking in persons report. June 2018. Available at: www.state.gov/documents/organization/282798.pdf. Accessed October 30, 2019.

Zimmerman C, Borland R (eds): Caring for trafficked persons: guidance for health providers. International Organization for Migration, 2009. Available at: https://publications.iom.int/system/files/pdf/ct_handbook.pdf. Accessed October 30, 2019.

CHAPTER 6

Managing Trafficked Persons With Comorbid Medical Conditions

Rachel Robitz, M.D.
Amy Gajaria, M.D., FRCPC

> When I start worrying about the future, I remind
> myself that we've got to live one day at a time.
>
> —*Carolyn, Peer educator*

A 32-year-old female with a past psychiatric history of bipolar disorder presents to a walk-in psychiatric clinic. She reports that she recently moved to a rural area with a friend because it was less expensive to live there. Initially, things went well, but then the people she was living with forced her to assist in the packaging of illicit drugs. She was also sexually assaulted several times. When she decided to leave the rural area to return to the city, she was told by the people she was living with that she could not. She did not have access to transportation, and her location was very remote. She ran out of her psychiatric medication, but she was not permitted by the people she was living with to visit a physician to get a refill of her medications. She eventually escaped and made her way to the nearest city. When she arrived, however, she had no housing and as a result had to sleep on the street. At today's visit, she reports not only that she is experiencing worsening depressive symptoms but also that she also has right wrist pain, chronic back pain, and pelvic pain. She also reports that on the day prior to the assessment she was sexually assaulted while sleeping on the street.

Individuals trafficked for both sex and labor, such as the individual in the above case example, are affected by a variety of health conditions. As a mental health provider, it is important to have an understanding of the common physical concerns of trafficked individuals, as these may impact an individual's mental health and/or his or her ability to engage in mental health treatment. In this chapter, we provide an overview of the health needs of both adults and minors who have been trafficked for labor and sex, and then we discuss a mental health provider's role in addressing these needs. We discuss common barriers to accessing medical care and how a mental health provider may help engage trafficked individuals in medical care. Because many trafficked individuals have comorbid medical and mental health conditions, mental health providers must work across disciplines to care for the complex needs of these vulnerable patients.

ADULTS

Common Medical Conditions

Literature about health conditions experienced by trafficked adults is somewhat limited. Much of the literature is internationally focused or focused on sex trafficking of women. There is limited domestic literature about labor trafficking and trafficking of men and transgender and gender nonconforming individuals. Much of the information presented here is derived from international data.

Domestically, trafficked individuals see a variety of health care providers while being trafficked. More than half of trafficked individuals receive care in emergency/urgent care settings, more than 40% see a primary care physician, and roughly a quarter see dentists and OB-GYNs (Chisolm-Straker et al. 2016). As demonstrated by the diversity of settings in which trafficked individuals are seen, they experience a broad range of both acute and chronic medical concerns. These conditions are a result of experiences of violence and trauma, poor working conditions, and poor living conditions (Table 6–1).

Because of their exposure to violence, trafficked individuals are at increased risk of traumatic injuries, including broken bones, head trauma, and stab wounds (Muftić and Finn 2013; Oram et al. 2016; Zimmerman 2007). Moreover, trafficked individuals may present late to care for these injuries (Baldwin et al. 2011). Delayed presentation of traumatic injuries for care can result in long-term sequelae, including chronic pain, mobility limitations, permanent scarring, and infection.

Along with these traumatic injuries, trafficked individuals are exposed to sexual violence (Ottisova et al. 2016; Zimmerman 2007). Mental health providers may consider referring trafficked individuals who present within 72 hours of a sexual assault for a forensic sex-

TABLE 6–1. Common medical conditions by exposure

	POOR WORKING CONDITIONS	POOR LIVING CONDITIONS	EXPOSURE TO PHYSICAL/SEXUAL VIOLENCE	EXPOSURE TO EMOTIONAL TRAUMA
Labor trafficking	Overuse injuries, exposure to chemicals, traumatic injuries	Malnutrition, skin conditions, dental disease	Traumatic injuries, sexually transmitted diseases, pelvic pain	Headaches, fatigue, dizziness, stomach pain
Sex trafficking	Sexually transmitted infections, pelvic pain	Malnutrition, skin conditions, dental disease	Traumatic injuries, sexually transmitted diseases, pelvic pain	Headaches, fatigue, dizziness, stomach pain

ual assault exam if the individual is agreeable. A *forensic sexual assault exam* is an exam to collect evidence to assist in prosecution of the perpetrator (Alempijevic et al. 2007). Often during these exams, the sexual assault victim is also offered postexposure prophylaxis to prevent sexually transmitted infections (STIs) as well as unwanted pregnancy (Alempijevic et al. 2007; Workowski and Berman 2002). The process of obtaining these exams varies by location, so providers should be knowledgeable about their local resources. If the assault occurred more than 72 hours earlier, mental health providers may consider referring the individual to a medical provider for STI testing and treatment.

Many of the medical conditions experienced by trafficked individuals are related to poor working conditions. For labor-trafficked individuals, these conditions vary based on the industry into which they are trafficked. In industries with repetitive physical labor such as domestic work, construction, agriculture, restaurants, hotels, and factory work, trafficked individuals may experience overuse injuries such as tendonitis and muscular strain (Ronda-Pérez and Moen 2017; Zimmerman et al. 2011). Overuse injuries can have prolonged treatment courses and at times be chronic with a relapsing and remitting course. Treatment often includes physical and occupational therapy. Individuals trafficked for agriculture, domestic work, hotel work, and restaurant work may be exposed to chemicals such as pesticides and cleaning solutions, which can result in long-term medical complications (Ronda-Pérez and Moen 2017; Zimmerman 2007; Zimmerman et al. 2011). Work-related injuries such as amputations, cuts, and broken bones caused by the limited use of personal protective equipment can occur in factory settings, construction, and agriculture (Ronda-Pérez and Moen 2017; Zimmerman et al. 2011). Similar to individuals with traumatic injuries that result from violence, persons with traumatic injuries due to poor working conditions may not seek medical care right away (Baldwin et al. 2011). It may be that care is not sought unless the injury results in an inability to work. Individuals trafficked for sex are at risk for STIs and pelvic pain (Muftić and Finn 2013; Zimmerman et al. 2008).

Along with conditions related to poor working environments, trafficked individuals are at increased risk because of poor living environments. Trafficked individuals may have little control over what and when they eat, so they may present with malnutrition (Muftić and Finn 2013; Zimmerman et al. 2011). Along with poor nutrition, they may have the inability to engage in dental hygiene and may be at increased risk of traumatic dental injuries. This can result in tooth pain in addition to other dental impairments (O'Callaghan 2012; Oram et al. 2012b). Poor nutrition can result in vitamin deficiencies that have consequential psychiatric symptoms. Moreover, providers, particularly on inpatient units, should be aware of the potential for refeeding syndrome (Catani and Howells 2007; Solomon and Kirby 1990).

Many trafficked individuals have a large spectrum of symptoms that may be related to poor working conditions, living conditions, and traumatic injuries, which may also overlap with the somatic symptoms seen with depression, anxiety, and somatic symptom disorders. More than half of trafficked individuals report symptoms such as headaches, stomach pain, and memory problems (Oram et al. 2012a, 2016; Ottisova et al. 2016; Zimmerman et al. 2008). Other common symptoms include back pain, fatigue, and dizziness (Oram et al. 2012a, 2012b; Ottisova et al. 2016; Zimmerman et al. 2008). Careful medical evaluation is necessary to evaluate for an underlying physiological cause of symptoms prior to attributing the symptoms to sequelae of emotional distress.

Barriers to Care

Much of the literature related to barriers to medical care discusses barriers to identification. Some literature, however, explores difficulties experienced by clinicians when providing medical care to trafficked persons. Trafficked individuals have been noted to have unique needs, and at times it is difficult to find appropriate providers with knowledge of how to work with trafficked individuals in a trauma-informed manner (Clawson and Dutch 2008). A study of sex-trafficked individuals (Ravi et al. 2017) found that these individuals sometimes feel intimidated when seeking medical care. They also express concerns that health care providers prioritize ability to pay over providing appropriate care (Ravi et al. 2017). Trafficked individuals want providers who are nonjudgmental and are able to communicate compassion and empathy (Ravi et al. 2017).

CHILDREN AND ADOLESCENTS

Common Medical Conditions

Literature related to trafficked individuals younger than 18 years has primarily focused on sex trafficking to the exclusion of labor trafficking, particularly when the focus is on domestically trafficked minors in the United States. The definition of human trafficking with respect to involvement in the commercial sex industry includes both children and youth younger than 18 who have been recruited and forced into the sex trade as well as youth engaged in commercial sex for other reasons. As a result, the literature regarding physical health consequences for trafficked young people does not differentiate between the health needs of young people engaged in the sex trade against their will and young people engaged in commercial sex voluntarily, and it is not known whether the health needs of these two populations vary.

That being said, there are many similarities in the health needs of pediatric trafficked individuals and the health needs of individuals over the age of 18. Literature on pediatric trafficked individuals has primarily focused on reproductive health, substance use, and mental health concerns, without focus on other areas of health that might be of concern to young trafficked individuals (Le et al. 2018). Finally, as in the adult population, the literature has also primarily focused on the health needs of young women in the sex trade, with limited research on the health needs of young men or transgender individuals (Greenbaum et al. 2015).

Trafficked young people experience similar health concerns to those older than 18. In particular, trafficked young women are also at elevated risk of physical injury due to an increased risk of violence that is part of the everyday existence of young women in the sex trade (Greenbaum et al. 2015; Young Women's Empowerment Project 2009). Malnutrition due to either restriction of oral intake by traffickers and/or the presence of comorbid disordered eating is also of significant concern, although there has been limited research specifically addressing malnutrition in trafficked individuals younger than age 18 (Le et al. 2018; West Coast Children's Clinic 2012). Issues of malnutrition in young trafficked individuals are of importance to those providing psychiatric care because young people entering inpatient or residential care environments may be at risk for refeeding syndrome. Malnourished young people may also have deficiencies in vitamin B_{12} or iron deficiency anemia, which may affect their psychiatric manifestations. In addition, the rates of disordered eating are higher in commercially sexually exploited youth, and thus mental health providers should screen for the presence of eating disorders and their medical complications when working with trafficked young people.

With respect to reproductive health issues, research has primarily focused on the needs of female trafficked individuals, although there is some evidence that trafficked young males may have higher rates of HIV infection (Le et al. 2018). Young trafficked individuals may have even higher rates of STIs, including HIV, particularly if they began trading sex as adolescents (Le et al. 2018). Trafficked adolescents also have higher rates of pregnancy-related complications, both for the adolescents and for their infants, when compared with adults or pregnant adolescents not engaged in the sex trade (Le et al. 2018; Willis and Levy 2002). Trafficked youth may also be at higher risk for cervical cancer, given the higher risk for HPV infection and decreased access to preventive health care (Le et al. 2018; Willis and Levy 2002).

Trafficked adolescents may not be up to date on their routine immunizations, particularly those vaccinations provided in adolescence (Greenbaum et al. 2015). Trafficked adolescents have higher rates of presenting with somatic complaints such as headaches, stomachaches, and dizziness (Ottisova et al. 2018; Zimmerman and Borland 2009). Given the high rates of physical violence experienced by these youth along with the other adverse consequences of poor living conditions, it can be challenging for mental health providers to differentiate between somatic presentations of distress and underlying health problems in trafficked adolescents.

Barriers to Care

Caring effectively for trafficked adolescents presents many challenges. Trafficked adolescents often have experienced violence from their caregivers prior to being trafficked, as well as repeated experiences of violence throughout their trafficking experience. Consequently, trafficked adolescents often have great challenges trusting new people and engaging in services (Clawson and Dutch 2008; Varma et al. 2015). Trafficked adolescents also report being wary of accessing both medical and mental health care because of fear of being judged by providers, fear of the police becoming involved (either for their current difficulties or for being arrested for previous charges), and fear that their concerns will not be kept confidential (Ijadi-Maghsoodi et al. 2018). Young trafficked transgender females express particular difficulty accessing health services because of fears that services will not be trans positive and because of repeated negative experiences with formal services and with police.

From a systems perspective, trafficked adolescents often struggle to access resources because of fragmentation in the sectors serving adolescents. In certain regions, if exploitation was not at the hands of a parent or guardian, child welfare agencies may not see serving these youth as part of their mandate (Clawson and Dutch 2008). In addition, trafficked youth have often been out of the formal education sector, lack stable housing, and lack a "point person" to help coordinate their care (Clawson and Dutch 2008; West Coast Children's Clinic 2012).

MENTAL HEALTH PROVIDER'S ROLE IN ADDRESSING MEDICAL NEEDS

Mental health providers must first have an awareness of the various health conditions that affect trafficked individuals. It is important to recognize whether an individual is currently being exploited, is early in his or her postexploitation recovery, or has been in a postexploitation stage for a longer period of time. Services should be targeted to the individual's needs as well as his or her current stage (i.e., current exploitation, early postexploitation recovery, postexploitation recovery). For example, whereas addressing immediate safety concerns is often the primary focus of services for individuals who are currently being exploited or are early in their postexploitation recovery, an individual further into their recovery may need a stronger focus on recovery from chronic conditions to improve functioning.

When working with currently exploited individuals, clinicians must first recognize what the limitations are in the ability of a trafficked individual's ability to care for his or her health. They likely have limited control over their ability to negotiate for their safety. For example, it may be difficult for a labor-trafficked individual to access personal protective equipment or for a sex-trafficked individual to negotiate condom usage. The trafficked individual likely knows far better than their provider what their safety needs are. Any discussion of preventive interventions should use a shared decision-making approach that allows the trafficked individual and provider to work in a collaborative manner to come up with a plan for safety and prevention.

The ideal situation for an individual's health and safety is to leave exploitation; however, not all trafficked individuals will be willing or ready to leave initially. If a trafficked individual is ready to leave, a clinician should help prevent further negative health consequences by working with local resources to help develop a safe exit plan. If an individual is not yet ready to leave their exploitive situation, a mental health provider may consider providing resources such as the National Human Trafficking Hotline number (1-888-373-7888) for use if they decide to leave in the future. Providers may also consider having condoms in their office. They should be aware of appropriate medical resources in their community, including urgent care services for the acute needs of labor- and sex-trafficked individuals and, particularly, family planning and sexual health resources for sex-trafficked individuals. Mental health providers working with trafficked individuals who are currently being trafficked and are not ready to leave may also consider doing safety planning with the individuals they serve. For example, the provider may help a trafficked individual learn how to identify objects in their environment that can be used for self-protection if one of their traffickers becomes violent.

For providers working with individuals in the posttrafficking stage, the care moves beyond addressing acute issues and risk reduction to assisting trafficked individuals in engaging in ongoing medical care for treatment of chronic conditions and basic preventive care. An integrated care approach in which behavioral health providers and primary care physicians work together to address a trafficked individual's needs is critical (Gordon et al. 2018). Mental health providers can provide consultation to primary care physicians, who may have limited training in how to work with individuals with significant trauma (Green et al. 2011). Moreover, collaborative care is important for addressing symptoms that sit at the interface of medical and psychiatric problems. For example, acceptance and commitment therapy is effective for chronic pain, and cognitive-behavioral therapy is effective for insomnia (Taylor and Pruiksma 2014; Veehof et al. 2011). Mental health providers may be critical partners with primary care providers in helping patients improve sleep, decrease chronic pain, practice healthy eating, regain healthy sexual functioning, and reduce smoking and other substance use that leads to poor health.

SPECIAL CONSIDERATIONS FOR WORKING WITH ADOLESCENTS

The best approach to ensuring that adequate care is provided to trafficked adolescents would include an interdisciplinary, trauma-informed, and strengths-based approach in which trafficked adolescents would be able to access services for their physical and mental health needs in one location (Steiner et al. 2018). Trafficked adolescents also benefit from having a primary point person, such as a case manager, who can help coordinate services for them, who can flexibly meet them where they're at, and who can access community-based services (Clawson and Dutch 2008; Ijadi-Maghsoodi et al. 2018;

West Coast Children's Clinic 2012). Such an approach would allow mental health providers to collaborate with primary care providers to address the places of overlap between mental health and physical health problems in this high-needs population.

CONCLUSION

Both adults and minors trafficked for labor and sex experience a variety of medical conditions that may complicate their mental health presentation and/or prevent them from fully engaging in mental health treatment. Understanding the common medical conditions that impact trafficked individuals can best help mental health providers to collaborate across disciplines to address the complex and unique needs of the individuals they serve.

Pearls and Pointers

- Individuals who have been trafficked experience a wide range of health conditions related to their exposure to violence and emotional trauma, poor working conditions, and poor living conditions.
- Mental health providers working with trafficked individuals should have an awareness of the common conditions experienced by this population and be knowledgeable about local community resources for addressing the needs of trafficked individuals.
- Coordination of services among physical and behavioral health providers is important for addressing the unique and complex needs of trafficked individuals.
- Individuals who are currently being trafficked may have needs that are more related to acute care, immediate safety, and risk reduction.

REFERENCES

Alempijevic D, Jecmenica D, Pavlekic S, et al: Forensic medical examination of victims of trafficking in human beings. Torture 17(2):117–121, 2007 17728488

Baldwin SB, Eisenman DP, Sayles JN, et al: Identification of human trafficking victims in health care settings. Health Hum Rights 13(1):E36–E49, 2011 22772961

Catani M, Howells R: Risks and pitfalls for the management of refeeding syndrome in psychiatric patients. Psychiatric Bulletin 31(6):209–211, 2007

Chisolm-Straker M, Baldwin S, Gaïgbé-Togbé B, et al: Health care and human trafficking: we are seeing the unseen. J Health Care Poor Underserved 27(3):1220–1233, 2016 27524764

Clawson HJ, Dutch N: Addressing the Needs of Victims of Human Trafficking: Challenges, Barriers, and Promising Practices. Washington, DC, Department of Health and Human Services, Office of the Assistant Secretary for Planning and Evaluation, 2008

Gordon M, Salami T, Coverdale J, et al: Psychiatry's role in the management of human trafficking victims: an integrated care approach. J Psychiatr Pract 24(2):79–86, 2018 29509177

Green BL, Kaltman SI, Frank L, et al: Primary care providers' experiences with trauma patients: a qualitative study. Psychol Trauma 3(1):37–41, 2011

Greenbaum J, Crawford-Jakubiak JE; Committee on Child Abuse and Neglect: Child sex trafficking and commercial sexual exploitation: health care needs of victims. Pediatrics 135(3):566–574, 2015 25713283

Ijadi-Maghsoodi R, Bath E, Cook M, et al: Commercially sexually exploited youths' health care experiences, barriers, and recommendations: a qualitative analysis. Child Abuse Negl 76:334–341, 2018 29195171

Le PD, Ryan N, Rosenstock Y, et al: Health issues associated with commercial sexual exploitation and sex trafficking of children in the United States: a systematic review. Behav Med 44(3):219–233, 2018 30020867

Muftić LR, Finn MA: Health outcomes among women trafficked for sex in the United States: a closer look. J Interpers Violence 28(9):1859–1885, 2013 23295378

O'Callaghan MG: Human trafficking and the dental professional. J Am Dent Assoc 143(5):498–504, 2012 22547722

Oram S, Ostrovschi NV, Gorceag VI, et al: Physical health symptoms reported by trafficked women receiving post-trafficking support in Moldova: prevalence, severity and associated factors. BMC Womens Health 12(1):20, 2012a 22834807

Oram S, Stöckl H, Busza J, et al: Prevalence and risk of violence and the physical, mental, and sexual health problems associated with human trafficking: systematic review. PLoS Med 9(5):e1001224, 2012b 22666182

Oram S, Abas M, Bick D, et al: Human trafficking and health: a survey of male and female survivors in England. Am J Public Health 106(6):1073–1078, 2016 27077341

Ottisova L, Hemmings S, Howard LM, et al: Prevalence and risk of violence and the mental, physical and sexual health problems associated with human trafficking: an updated systematic review. Epidemiol Psychiatr Sci 25(4):317–341, 2016 27066701

Ottisova L, Smith P, Oram S: Psychological consequences of human trafficking: complex posttraumatic stress disorder in trafficked children. Behav Med 44(3):234–241, 2018 30020865

Ravi A, Pfeiffer MR, Rosner Z, et al: Identifying health experiences of domestically sex-trafficked women in the USA: a qualitative study in Rikers Island jail. J Urban Health 94(3):408–416, 2017 28116589

Ronda-Pérez E, Moen BE: Labour trafficking: Challenges and opportunities from an occupational health perspective. PLoS Med 14(11):e1002440, 2017 29166395

Solomon SM, Kirby DF: The refeeding syndrome: a review. JPEN J Parenter Enteral Nutr 14(1):90–97, 1990 2109122

Steiner JJ, Kynn J, Stylianou AM, et al: Providing services to trafficking survivors: understanding practices across the globe. J Evid Inf Soc Work 15(2):150–168, 2018 29336727

Taylor DJ, Pruiksma KE: Cognitive and behavioural therapy for insomnia (CBT-I) in psychiatric populations: a systematic review. Int Rev Psychiatry 26(2):205–213, 2014 24892895

Varma S, Gillespie S, McCracken C, et al: Characteristics of child commercial sexual exploitation and sex trafficking victims presenting for medical care in the United States. Child Abuse Negl 44:98–105, 2015 25896617

Veehof MM, Oskam MJ, Schreurs KM, et al: Acceptance-based interventions for the treatment of chronic pain: a systematic review and meta-analysis. Pain 152(3):533–542, 2011 21251756

West Coast Children's Clinic: Research to Action: Sexually Exploited Minors Needs and Strengths. Oakland, CA, 2012

Willis BM, Levy BS: Child prostitution: global health burden, research needs, and interventions. Lancet 359(9315):1417–1422, 2002 11978356

Workowski KA, Berman SM: CDC sexually transmitted diseases treatment guidelines. Clin Infect Dis 35(Suppl 2):S135–S137, 2002 12353199

Young Women's Empowerment Project: Girls do what they have to do to survive: illuminating methods used by girls in the sex trade and street economy to fight back and heal. 2009. Available at: https://ywep-chicago.files.wordpress.com/2011/06/girls-do-what-they-have-to-do-to-survive-a-study-of-resilience-and-resistance.pdf. Accessed October 29, 2019.

Zimmerman C: Trafficking in women: the health of women in post-trafficking services in Europe who were trafficked into prostitution or sexually abused as domestic labourers. PhD Thesis, London School of Hygiene and Tropical Medicine, 2007. Available at: https://pdfs.semanticscholar.org/436e/8f967daeef330887643f1accedfafdb37178.pdf?_ga=2.151305977.1314921934.1572460066-586094439.1572460066. Accessed October 30, 2019.

Zimmerman C, Borland R (eds): Caring for trafficked persons: guidance for health providers. International Organization for Migration, 2009. Available at: https://publications.iom.int/system/files/pdf/ct_handbook.pdf. Accessed October 30, 2019.

Zimmerman C, Hossain M, Yun K, et al: The health of trafficked women: a survey of women entering posttrafficking services in Europe. Am J Public Health 98(1):55–59, 2008 18048781

Zimmerman C, Hossain M, Watts C: Human trafficking and health: a conceptual model to inform policy, intervention and research. Soc Sci Med 73(2):327–335, 2011 21723653

General Principles of Care for Trafficked Persons

Kimberly S. G. Chang, M.D., M.P.H.

Robert P. Marlin, M.D., Ph.D., M.P.H.

> Of all the forms of inequality, injustice in health is the most shocking and inhuman…
>
> —*Martin Luther King Jr.*[1]

A 34-year-old female Chinese immigrant who was sex trafficked and has an open legal case against the traffickers is receiving advocacy services from a local nongovernmental organization in the county in which she was sex trafficked. The case manager notes that the client does not trust any professionals and refuses to leave her apartment. She has been eating only ramen noodles, which are stacked up to the ceiling in her apartment, because of her fear of being poisoned by her traffickers. The case manager notes that the client should receive medical and mental health evaluations. However, her Medicaid coverage is tied to her residence in another county. As a result, the case manager must refer her for medical care to the community health center in the county of her residence. The client is referred to the community health center's specialty mental health unit to be evaluated.

Human trafficking is legislatively defined both in the United States (Trafficking Victims Protection Act of 2000 [P.L. 106-386]) and internationally as a crime; human trafficking might also be described as a health hazard, because there is recognition by the federal government that human trafficking results in severe health consequences affecting some of the most vulnerable members of society (Chon 2015). Short- and long-term health harms are caused by the conditions of human trafficking and the manner in which people

---

[1]Quoted in Galarneau 2018.

are controlled for labor or sex. While trafficked, people are frequently deprived of health care and food; socially restricted; coerced into substance use and dependence; forced into dangerous, dirty, and degrading living and working conditions; and subjected to physical, sexual, psychological, emotional, behavioral, and spiritual abuse (Baldwin et al. 2011). These health harms fall into three categories: 1) physical harms, such as sexually transmitted infections, injuries, and malnutrition; 2) mental health harms, such as trauma, depression, and anxiety; and 3) social harms, such as criminalization and stigmatization (Baldwin et al. 2011; Crane and Moreno 2011; Dovydaitis 2010; Felitti et al. 1998; Institute of Medicine and National Research Council 2013; Isaac et al. 2011; Willis and Levy 2002; Zimmerman et al. 2003). In addition to care for these acute and long-term health harmful effects, trafficked persons need primary care, just like other patients. A primary care approach emphasizes prevention, community outreach, and multidisciplinary collaboration, with a focus on addressing social determinants of health and preventing harm (Todres 2011). Any clinician caring for a trafficked person should always ensure that the patient is connected to a primary care provider.

Because of the conditions of violence and exploitation under which they live or have lived, special considerations are required in the care for trafficked persons; trafficked persons have specific health care needs as a result of their status. However, they are still patients with many of the same fundamental care needs, complaints, and concerns as most other patients. Health care providers need to exercise caution and not automatically assume that all complaints relate to their history of human trafficking. At the same time, many clinical conditions in trafficked persons may be more advanced as trafficked persons may not have had regular access to primary care. In this chapter, we address general primary care principles that behavioral health clinicians should consider in the cases of trafficked persons and those special populations at risk of being trafficked.

HEALTH CARE ACCESS AND COVERAGE

Despite the clear need for services, trafficked persons face multiple barriers to accessing primary care. A large proportion are unauthorized immigrants who do not qualify for state or federally funded health care coverage (American Civil Liberties Union 2019). Six states (California, Illinois, Massachusetts, New York, Oregon, and

Washington) and the District of Columbia have expanded Medicaid programs that insure all income-eligible children, regardless of immigration status (Henry J. Kaiser Family Foundation 2019b; National Conference of State Legislatures 2017). Massachusetts also offers health care coverage for unauthorized, income-eligible adults at acute care hospitals and community health centers (Commonwealth of Massachusetts 2019). Some states will also cover pregnancy-related health care services for undocumented immigrants (Henry J. Kaiser Family Foundation 2019a). Individuals in other states who are uninsured can still access primary care services at federally qualified health centers (Table 7–1), regardless of insurance or immigration status (Health Center Program Statute 2019). Even in states that do offer health care coverage for unauthorized immigrants or Medicaid to low-income residents who are not unauthorized immigrants, these individuals must still apply. This is where trafficked persons, both unauthorized immigrants and nonimmigrants, often encounter obstacles.

Many trafficked persons are wary of involvement with government entities or institutions because of fear of prosecution for criminal activity (Atkinson et al. 2016; Institute of Medicine and National Research Council 2013). Although many states have adopted "safe harbor" laws, which protect trafficked minors from being prosecuted for criminal activity and provide them with needed services, these vary from state to state and do not cover adults (Institute of Medicine and National Research Council 2013). Minors may not be aware of protections under these laws. Unauthorized immigrants also fear deportation if they declare themselves to any government-affiliated program. Many trafficked persons may also not have the identification or documents required to apply for health care coverage, such as a birth certificate, proof of income, or a social security number. Applicants also need to have a stable residential address at which they can receive confirmation of their coverage application or renewal notices by mail. Many trafficked persons may not have stable housing or may be homeless. Even when eligible, minors generally need to have a parent or legal guardian with them to apply for health care coverage, and trafficked youth will not have access to either (Halley and English 2008). Trafficked minors are generally not enrolled in school, where they might otherwise be able to access school-based health services without having to apply for coverage. In addition to being homeless, many trafficked persons are food insecure. When faced with real or perceived costs of primary care, such as copays,

TABLE 7–1. Federally Qualified Health Centers: finding a community health center

FINDING A COMMUNITY HEALTH CENTER NEAR YOU

This useful tool helps you find potential Federally Qualified Health Center primary care sites for your patients based on zip code: https://findahealthcenter.hrsa.gov/

Description

Health centers are consumer-driven and patient-centered organizations that serve as a comprehensive and cost-effective primary health care option for America's most underserved communities. Health centers serve everyone, regardless of ability to pay or insurance status. They increase access to health care and provide integrated services based on the unique needs of the communities they serve. There are four key components of health centers:

1. Located in high areas of need—designated as medically underserved areas or populations by the federal government

2. Comprehensive set of services—based on community needs, health centers offer medical, dental, vision, behavioral health, and enabling services

3. Open to everyone—regardless of insurance status or ability to pay, and offer sliding fee scale options to low-income patients

4. Patient-majority governing boards—at least 51% of every health center's governing board must be made up of patients

Source. Adapted from National Association of Community Health Centers 2018.

transportation, or prescription charges, they may opt instead to put whatever money they have toward food.

In addition to ensuring health insurance coverage and mitigating barriers to accessing health care, behavioral health clinicians should be aware of various health care access points and the need for continuity in primary care. Primary care practice settings include community health centers (e.g., migrant, public housing, and rural health centers) (Chang and Hayashi 2017), adolescent medicine clinics, school clinics, hospital-based primary care outpatient clinics, public health department clinics, free-standing Title X clinics, Planned Parenthood clinics, free clinics, and private practices (Cohen 2005; Institute of Medicine and National Research Council 2013). The Health Resources and Services Administration website Find a Health Center (available at https://findahealthcenter.hrsa.gov/) is a useful tool for finding a health center in the local area. Patients may also access health care in emergency departments, commercial urgent care clinics, or dental clinics (Chisolm-Straker et al. 2016). However, given the nature of the physical, mental health, and social harms that are characteristic of trafficked persons, it is imperative that patients are connected to primary care for close follow-up and wrap-around services.

LANGUAGE ACCESS

Providing access to professional medical interpreters is important for all patients with limited English proficiency, but such access is imperative for trafficked persons. Traffickers accompanying patients to clinical appointments may claim to be a relative or a friend and insist that the patient prefers to have them interpret rather than a professional interpreter. Most institutions and states have policies mandating that health care providers use professional interpreters with patients whose proficiency in English is limited, rather than friends or family members, and the National Standards for Culturally and Linguistically Appropriate Services in Health and Health Care of the U.S. Department of Health and Human Services support this (U.S. Department of Health and Human Services 2019). Insistence not to have a professional interpreter by someone accompanying a patient with limited English proficiency should serve as a red flag for the health care team to evaluate the patient for human trafficking. Clinicians and other team members should invoke these policies and standards and enlist the services of a professional medical interpreter. This also provides an opportunity to remove the accompanying person from the room so that the patient can be educated about and possibly assessed for human trafficking.

Medical interpreters who will be working with trafficked persons need to be trained in trauma-informed care practices, along with the rest of the care team. Whenever possible, they should be advised in advance when the clinician suspects exploitation or human trafficking so that they are prepared for emotionally difficult interactions. Their training should include how to manage vicarious trauma, as they will be voicing the words and the experiences of trafficked patients in the first person.

While face-to-face interpreting is generally preferred by most patients and clinicians, some trafficked persons from smaller linguistic communities may prefer to use telephonic or video interpretation. They may not feel secure speaking in front of someone from their local community, as opposed to speaking with an interpreter located in another state or region. Trafficked persons should be asked which mode of interpretation they prefer.

TRAUMA-INFORMED CONSIDERATIONS

An essential goal of primary care for trafficked persons must be to make them feel safe enough to initially engage in care and then continue in care, if possible. This is best accomplished through the adoption of a trauma-informed primary care model. Trauma-informed primary care is based on the realization that the experience of trauma, including human trafficking, is closely connected to subsequent illness and unhealthy behaviors. This paradigm recognizes trauma as an important social determinant of health (Machtinger et al. 2015). In trauma-informed primary care, clinical practices and policies are redesigned to accommodate the specific needs of trauma survivors.

Adopting this model of care benefits not only trafficked persons but other trauma survivors as well. There is a high rate of trauma among the U.S. primary care population generally, and clinicians will not necessarily be able to identify trafficked persons among their patients in advance (Mace and Smith 2019). Thus, adopting trauma-informed primary care practices and policies broadly will help make these patients more comfortable opening up to clinicians about their history and enlisting their help.

Unlike other trauma survivors, trafficked persons may engage in health care less frequently because of restrictions imposed by traffickers on their ability to access care and to have contact with other people. For this reason, it is essential that primary care teams be trained in trauma-informed primary care and prepared for the possibility of disclosure and identification of trafficked persons to ensure that these patients will not be retraumatized in the process of accessing health care (Mace and Smith 2019).

SAFETY PLANNING CONSIDERATIONS FOR PATIENTS

Safety planning is a crucial component of the patient visit and can occur during any of the three phases of being trafficked: while a patient may be experiencing trafficking, during the process of leaving a trafficking situation, and once the trafficked person has left the situation. Safety planning must be individualized; this can be accomplished with the clinician or other members of the care team, such as a case manager or mental health provider. It is paramount that the clinician acknowledge that the affected patient is in the best position to assess his or her safety level. According to the National Human Trafficking Hotline, safety planning can benefit patients during all phases of trafficking. Safety plans include risk assessments, preparations, and contingency plans:

1. Assess current risk; identify current and potential safety concerns.
2. Create strategies to avoid or reduce the threat of harm.
3. Outline concrete options for responding when safety is threatened or compromised.

The National Human Trafficking Hotline website (available at https://humantraffickinghotline.org/faqs/safety-planning-information) has useful tips for clinicians on safety assessment.

VACCINES

Trafficked persons require all recommended vaccinations based on age, as well as those based on specific medical conditions or risk factors. Updated vaccine schedules can be found at the Centers for Disease Control and Prevention's website (www.cdc.gov/vaccines/schedules/index.html). It is crucial that clinicians caring for trafficked persons provide this recommended and standard preventive care. Special consideration should be given to the Td/Tdap vaccines, given occupational safety hazards in exploitative situations. The human papillomavirus (HPV) vaccine series should be administered in patients up to age 26 years. The HPV vaccine has recently been approved by the FDA in patients up to age 45 years and should be considered in these adults, given the increased risk in trafficked individuals for exploitative, forced, or coerced sex and lack of agency in trafficking situations (U.S. Food and Drug Administration 2018). If immunity does not exist, hepatitis A and hepatitis B vaccine series should be administered to any trafficked person. Given the high risk of being retrafficked and the use of intravenous drugs as a coercive tool, protection against viral hepatitis is crucial. Behavioral health clinicians should not miss any opportunities to refer trafficked persons to clinicians and advocate that medical clinicians provide immunizations while waiting to connect the patient to a primary care home. This will ensure that patients catch up on their vaccine schedule to maximize protection against preventable infectious disease.

SCREENING AND DISEASE PREVENTION

All regular preventive primary care should be offered to trafficked patients. The U.S. Preventive Services Task Force (USPSTF) provides evidence-based recommendations and should be consulted regularly for updates to primary care practice (see appendix to this chapter). When considering screening and disease prevention in this population, it is important to consider the context of trafficking, lack of agency, experience of violence, and, if known, type of trafficking and trauma experienced by the patient. For example, the USPSTF has a Grade B recommendation for hepatitis B screening in persons at high risk of infection. Although "high-risk" populations are not specified in the guidelines, persons who have been trafficked should be considered high risk given the context of force, fraud, or coercion for labor or sex trafficking and lack of agency. Other preventive measures that have not yet been evaluated with a robust body of evidence but should be considered include anorectal cancer screening and pre-exposure prophylaxis for HIV.

CHRONIC DISEASE MANAGEMENT

Chronic diseases, such as asthma, diabetes, and hypertension, often go untreated in trafficked persons, in large part because of a lack of regular care but also because of a lack of access to medications. Without coverage in place, trafficked persons may not be able to access primary care and, therefore, prescriptions for chronic conditions. If these patients are able to obtain prescriptions without coverage, they will often pay high commercial prices for medications. The 340B Drug Pricing Program is a good source for lower-cost, subsidized prescription medications. These medications are made available at discounted rates through "covered entities" such as safety net hospitals and federally qualified health centers (Health Resources and Services Administration 2019). Chronic diseases among trafficking survivors may also be exacerbated by the occupational and environmental exposures to which these patients are subjected.

REPRODUCTIVE HEALTH

Close attention should be paid to reproductive health. The behavioral health clinician should consider reproductive health harms in both sex- and labor-trafficked individuals because of these patients' increased risk for sexual violence and reproductive coercion. Repeated sexual abuse, sexually transmitted infections, and a lack of access to contraception during trafficking are related to unwanted pregnancies and gynecological symptoms (Macias-Konstantopoulos and Ma 2017). Trafficked persons may be subjected to violent beatings to induce miscarriages, and the behavioral health clinician should consider that the patient may have long-term consequences from forced, unsafe abortions. In cases in which pregnant women and girls are allowed or made to carry their pregnancy to term, few may receive prenatal care (Macias-Konstantopoulos and Ma 2017).

INTEGRATION OF PRIMARY CARE AND BEHAVIORAL HEALTH

There is a movement to integrate primary care and behavioral health care. In 2005, the Institute of Medicine issued the seminal report "Improving the Quality of Health Care for Mental and Substance-Use Conditions," which established principles for such integration (Institute of Medicine et al. 2005). For trafficked persons, the conditions of exploitation, violence, and abuse are severe, affecting mood, cognition, behavior, and function, as well as physical conditions. Patients with mental/behavioral issues present to primary care providers with concerns relating to mood disorders, stress, relationship issues, cognitive difficulties, and daily functioning. In addition, these patients can face challenges as new immigrants or in adopting healthy lifestyles. Trafficked persons may also present with symptoms of severe mental illness.

The most important principle behind care integration is communication. Primary care providers may not be aware of the extent of trauma or mental health effects stemming from trafficking experiences, so it is critical that behavioral health clinicians highlight possible connections with patients' physical health, relational and behavioral issues, cognitive status, and ability to access resources, for example. Case management is essential to ensuring that trafficked patients can navigate systems of care and protection and access concrete resources essential to healing and thriving. Behavioral health clinicians can assist in building the capacity of primary care providers to care for patients who have undergone complex trauma.

There are three proposed frameworks for the integration of primary care with behavioral health care: 1) consultative/coordinated, 2) co-located, and 3) collaborative/integrated. In a consultative/coordinated framework, care occurs in separate physical spaces. In a co-located model, care is within the same office space but is managed separately. In a collaborative/integrated rubric, the behavioral health specialist provides case consultation on primary care patients and works closely with primary care providers and other primary care–based behavioral health providers. Whatever model is used, bidirectional communication should be emphasized, given the complexity of mental, behavioral, and physical health needs for trafficked patients. The Health Resources and Services Administration's Center for Integrated Health Solutions provides more information on models of care (www.integration.samhsa.gov/integrated-care-models/behavioral-health-in-primary-care).

SUBSTANCE USE DISORDERS

When assessing patients, the presence of any substance use disorder should be considered as a potential sign of trafficking (Lederer and Wetzel 2014). Traffickers may use a wide range of substances to control the behavior and actions of trafficked persons. At the same time, such use by trafficked persons on their own may represent a maladaptive coping mechanism. In either case, such substance use puts trafficked persons at high risk for being charged criminally, which could mean deportation for unauthorized immigrants (Wood 2018). Reduction and cessation can be achieved through regular visits with primary care team members.

LEGAL CONSIDERATIONS

Safe harbor laws in many states allow trafficked minors to safely disclose their histories and receive care and access to dedicated resources, rather than prosecution for criminal activities (Polaris 2015). Minors in states without such laws and adult trafficked persons throughout the United States often fear sharing their trafficking histories with clinicians (Atkinson et al. 2016). This is especially true for unauthorized immigrants, who justifiably fear that any contact with law enforcement could end in deportation to countries that they no longer know or where they could face an even greater risk of violence.

The Trafficking Victims Protection Act of 2000 does provide specific protections for unauthorized immigrant trafficked persons in the form of the T visa program. This program allows trafficked persons to legally remain in the United States and provides a path to permanent residence (Trafficking Victim Protection Act of 2000; P.L. 106-386). However, reaching these goals requires trafficked persons to engage in a long and arduous process that includes assisting law enforcement in the prosecution of their traffickers (U.S. Citizenship and Immigration Services 2018). Even when working with law enforcement agencies, trafficked persons have no right to legal assistance and continue to feel legally vulnerable (Polaris 2015). Although the U.S. government acknowledges that there are approximately 50,000 adults and minors trafficked into the country annually, the Trafficking Victims Protection Act of 2000 only allows for up to 5,000 T visas annually. This means that the vast majority of trafficked persons will not be eligible for this program and, therefore, fear disclosing their histories (Yoder 2011).

Access to safe, reliable legal services is essential for all trafficked persons, minors and adults, unauthorized immigrants and U.S. citizens alike. Even with legal protections in place, many are unaware of the existence of protections or their rights. Health care settings, including primary care clinics, are one of the few places where trafficked persons may have a chance to speak with someone alone about their trafficking history, without their traffickers present. For this reason, it is ideal if legal services for trafficked persons are co-located with primary care services and offered through collaborations between clinicians and attorneys. The clinical needs of these patients cannot usually be adequately addressed without providing them with access to housing, food, health care coverage, and occupational protections, all of which require legal interventions or assurances.

SPECIAL POPULATIONS

Because of media narratives, common misperceptions about who may be trafficked, or the marginalization of certain groups from the mainstream population, some populations may be more invisible. Additional thought and consideration should be paid to labor-trafficked individuals, men and boys, racial and ethnic minorities, LGBTQ individuals, American Indian and other indigenous people, immigrants and refugees of varying documentation status, individuals with severe mental illness, cognitively impaired individuals, and those with housing insecurity and instability.

Special considerations for patients who have experienced human trafficking are complex trauma, the possibility of strangulation, and traumatic brain injury as causes of emotional or behavioral changes. However, the clinician must rule out organic disease rather than assuming any signs or symptoms are the sequelae of trauma.

CONCLUSION

In this chapter, we address general primary care principles that behavioral health clinicians should consider for trafficked persons and those special populations of individuals at risk of being trafficked. When caring for patients who have experienced human trafficking, the behavioral health clinician should advocate for and connect the patient with primary care, where recommended preventive care services can be provided. Considerations for behavioral health clinicians include health care coverage and access to care, language access, trauma-informed care principles, safety planning, immunizations, recommended screening and preventive measures, chronic disease management, reproductive health, integration of primary and behavioral health care, substance use disorders, legal issues, and special populations. Awareness of the general principles of care for trafficked patients will enable the behavioral health clinician to accelerate healing for patients.

Pearls and Pointers

- The clinician's role is to provide quality health care to patients. Patient disclosure of exploitation or identification of human trafficking victimization is the goal of the criminal justice sector but not of health care professionals.

- A universal education approach is paramount before any "screening" takes place. There are no 100% sensitive or 100% specific screening tools or questions. Improving health, decreasing isolation, providing resources and education on rights, reframing the issue, and maximizing safety outcomes are the goals for health care professionals.

- Special considerations for patients who have experienced human trafficking are complex trauma, the possibility of strangulation, and traumatic brain injury as causes of emotional or behavioral changes. However, the clinician must rule out organic disease rather than assuming any signs or symptoms are the sequelae of trauma.

- Recommended preventive measures are the standard of care for patients who have experienced trafficking and exploitation. There may be special considerations, such as administration of the human papillomavirus vaccine in people ages 26–45 years.

- Any patient who is diagnosed with a substance use disorder should be assessed for a possible history of trafficking or trauma.

REFERENCES

American Civil Liberties Union: Human trafficking: modern enslavement of immigrant women in the United States. 2019. Available at: www.aclu.org/other/human-trafficking-modern-enslavement-immigrant-women-united-states. Accessed October 30, 2019.

Atkinson HG, Curnin KJ, Hanson NC: U.S. state laws addressing human trafficking: education of and mandatory reporting by health care providers and other professionals. Journal of Human Trafficking 2(2):111–138, 2016

Baldwin SB, Eisenman DP, Sayles JN, et al: Identification of human trafficking victims in health care settings. Health Hum Rights 13(1):E36–E49, 2011 22772961

Chang KSG, Hayashi AS: The role of community health centers in addressing human trafficking, in Human Trafficking Is a Public Health Issue: A Paradigm Expansion in the United States. Edited by Chisolm-Straker M, Stoklosa H. New York, Springer, 2017, pp 347–362

Chisolm-Straker M, Baldwin S, Gaïgbé-Togbé B, et al: Health care and human trafficking: we are seeing the unseen. J Health Care Poor Underserved 27(3):1220–1233, 2016 27524764

Chon K: The power of framing human trafficking as a public health issue. Office of Trafficking in Persons, Administration for Family and Children, U.S. Department of Health and Human Services. Remarks at the "Paths to Equity" Women's Funding Network. Adapted from October 7, 2015 speech. Available at: www.acf.hhs.gov/programs/endtrafficking/resource/publichealthlens. Accessed October 30, 2019.

Cohen SA: Ominous convergence: sex trafficking, prostitution and international family planning. Guttmacher Policy Review, February 5, 2005. Available at: www.guttmacher.org/gpr/2005/02/ominous-convergence-sex-trafficking-prostitution-and-international-family planning. Accessed October 30, 2019.

Commonwealth of Massachusetts: Eligibility for health care benefits for MassHealth, the Health Safety Net, and Children's Medical Security Plan. 2019. Available at: www.mass.gov/service-details/eligibility-for-health-care-benefits-for-masshealth-the-health-safety-net-and. Accessed October 30, 2019.

Crane P, Moreno M: Human trafficking: what is the role of the health care provider? Journal of Applied Research on Children 2(1):1–27, 2011

Dovydaitis T: Human trafficking: the role of the health care provider. J Midwifery Womens Health 55(5):462–467, 2010 20732668

Felitti VJ, Anda RF, Nordenberg D, et al: Relationship of childhood abuse and household dysfunction to many of the leading causes of death in adults. The Adverse Childhood Experiences (ACE) Study. Am J Prev Med 14(4):245–258, 1998 9635069

Galarneau C: Getting King's words right. J Health Care Poor Underserved 29(1):5–8, 2018 29503282

Halley M, English A: Health care for homeless youth: policy options for improving access. Center for Adolescent Health and the Law; Public Policy Analysis and Education Center for Middle Childhood, Adolescent, and Young Adult Health, 2008. Available at: http://nahic.ucsf.edu/wp-content/uploads/2009/02/2009-Homeless-Brief.pdf. Accessed October 30, 2019.

Health Center Program Statute: Section 330 of the Public Health Service Act (42 U.S.C. §254b). October 30, 2019. Available at: https://uscode.house.gov/view.xhtml?req=granuleid:USC-prelim-title42-section254b&num=0&edition=prelim. Accessed October 30, 2019.

Health Resources and Services Administration: 340B drug pricing program. August 2019. Available at: www.hrsa.gov/opa/index.html. Accessed October 30, 2019.

Henry J. Kaiser Family Foundation: Health coverage of immigrants. February 15, 2019a. Available at: www.kff.org/disparities-policy/fact-sheet/health-coverage-of-immigrants/. Accessed October 30, 2019.

Henry J. Kaiser Family Foundation: Status of state action on the Medicaid expansion decision. 2019b. Available at: www.kff.org/health-reform/state-indicator/state-activity-around-expanding-medicaid-under-the-affordable-care-act/?currentTimeframe=0andsort-Model=%7B%22colId%22:%22Location%22,%22sort%22:%22asc%22%7D. Accessed October 30, 2019.

Institute of Medicine, National Research Council: Confronting Commercial Sexual Exploitation and Sex Trafficking of Minors in the United States. Washington, DC, National Academies Press, 2013

Institute of Medicine; Board on Health Care Services; Committee on Crossing the Quality Chasm: Adaptation to Mental Health and Addictive Disorders. Improving the Quality of Health Care for Mental and Substance-Use Conditions: Quality Chasm Series. Washington, DC, National Academies Press, 2005

Isaac R, Solak J, Giardino A: Health care providers' training needs related to human trafficking: maximizing the opportunity to effectively screen and intervene. Journal of Applied Research on Children 2(1):1–33, 2011

Lederer LJ, Wetzel CA: The health consequences of sex trafficking and their implications for identifying victims in healthcare facilities. Annals of Health Law 23(1):61–91, 2014

Mace S, Smith R: Trauma-informed care in primary care: a literature review. Kaiser Permanente and the National Council for Behavioral Health, 2019. Available at: www.nationalcouncildocs.net/wp-content/

uploads/2018/07/Trauma-Informed-Care-for-Primary-Care-Literature-Review.pdf. Accessed October 30, 2019.

Machtinger EL, Cuca YP, Khanna N, et al: From treatment to healing: the promise of trauma-informed primary care. Womens Health Issues 25(3):193–197, 2015 25965151

Macias-Konstantopoulos W, Ma ZB: Physical health of human trafficking survivors: unmet essentials, in Human Trafficking Is a Public Health Issue: A Paradigm Expansion in the United States. Edited by Chisolm-Straker M, Stoklosa H. New York, Springer, 2017, pp 185–210

National Association of Community Health Centers: America's Health Centers. August 2018. Available at: www.nachc.org/wp-content/uploads/2018/08/AmericasHealthCenters_FINAL.pdf.

National Conference of State Legislatures: Immigrant eligibility for health care programs in the United Sates. October 19, 2017. Available at: www.ncsl.org/research/immigration/immigrant-eligibility-for-health-care-programs-in-the-united-states.aspx. Accessed October 30, 2019.

Polaris: Human trafficking issue brief: safe harbor. 2015. Available at: https://polarisproject.org/sites/default/files/2015%20Safe%20Harbor%20Issue%20Brief.pdf. Accessed October 30, 2019.

Todres J: Moving upstream: the merits of a public health law approach to human trafficking. Georgia State University College of Law, Legal Studies Research Paper No. 2011-02. 89 N.C. L. REV. 447. The Social Science Research Network Electro Paper Collection. 2011. Available at: http://ssrn.com/abstract=1742953. Accessed October 30, 2016.

Trafficking Victims Protection Act of 2000, Pub. L. No. 106-386 (22 U.S.C. §78). Available at: https://uscode.house.gov/view.xhtml?path=/prelim@title22/chapter78andedition=prelim. Accessed October 30, 2019.

U.S. Citizenship and Immigration Services: Victims of human trafficking: T nonimmigrant status. May 10, 2018. Available at: www.uscis.gov/humanitarian/victims-human-trafficking-other-crimes/victims-human-trafficking-t-nonimmigrant-status. Accessed October 30, 2019.

U.S. Department of Health and Human Services: National culturally and linguistically appropriate service standards. 2019. Available at: www.thinkculturalhealth.hhs.gov/clas/standards. Accessed October 30, 2019.

U.S. Food and Drug Administration: FDA approves expanded use of Gardasil 9 to include individuals 27 through 45 years old. October 5, 2018. Available at: www.fda.gov/news-events/press-announcements/fda-approves-expanded-use-gardasil-9-include-individuals-27-through-45-years-old. Accessed October 30, 2019.

Willis BM, Levy BS: Child prostitution: global health burden, research needs, and interventions. Lancet 359(9315):1417–1422, 2002 11978356

Wood SP: The intersection of human trafficking and immigration. Petrie-Flom Center for Health Law Policy, Biotechnology, and Bioethics at Harvard Law School, June 27, 2018. Available at: http://blog.petrieflom.law.harvard.edu/2018/06/27/the-intersection-of-human-trafficking-and-immigration/. Accessed October 30, 2019.

Yoder HA: Civil rights for victims of human trafficking. University of Pennsylvania Journal of Law and Social Change, 2011. Available at: https://scholarship.law.upenn.edu/jlasc/vol12/iss2/1/. Accessed October 30, 2019.

Zimmerman C, Yun K, Shvab I, et al: The health risks and consequences of trafficking in women and adolescents: findings from a European study. London School of Hygiene and Tropical Medicine, 2003. Available at: https://researchonline.lshtm.ac.uk/id/eprint/10786. Accessed October 30, 2019.

APPENDIX:
SAMPLE USPSTF SCREENING RECOMMENDATIONS WITH SPECIAL CONSIDERATIONS FOR PATIENTS WITH A HISTORY OF BEING TRAFFICKED

USPSTF GRADE DEFINITIONS (AFTER JULY 2012)

A	The USPSTF recommends the service. There is high certainty that the net benefit is substantial. Offer or provide this service.
B	The USPSTF recommends the service. There is high certainty that the net benefit is moderate or there is moderate certainty that the net benefit is moderate to substantial. Offer or provide this service.
C	The USPSTF recommends selectively offering or providing this service to individual patients based on professional judgment and patient preferences. There is at least moderate certainty that the net benefit is small. Offer or provide this service for selected patients depending on individual circumstances.
D	The USPSTF recommends against the service. There is moderate or high certainty that the service has no net benefit or that the harms outweigh the benefits. Discourage the use of this service.
I statement	The USPSTF concludes that the current evidence is insufficient to assess the balance of benefits and harms of the service. Evidence is lacking, of poor quality, or conflicting, and the balance of benefits and harms cannot be determined. Read the clinical considerations section of USPSTF Recommendation Statement. If the service is offered, patients should understand the uncertainty about the balance of benefits and harms.

APPENDIX. Sample United States Preventive Services Task Force (USPSTF) screening recommendations with special considerations for patients with a history of being trafficked

ISSUE AREA	POPULATION	RECOMMENDATION	GRADE	CONSIDERATIONS IN HUMAN TRAFFICKING
Depression in adults: screening	General adult population, including pregnant and postpartum women	The USPSTF recommends screening for depression in the general adult population, including pregnant and postpartum women. Screening should be implemented with adequate systems in place to ensure accurate diagnosis, effective treatment, and appropriate follow-up.	B	Long-term mental health harms, including depression, affect survivors of human trafficking and should be screened for and addressed if present.
Gynecological conditions: periodic screening with the pelvic examination	Asymptomatic, nonpregnant adult women who are not at increased risk for any specific gynecologic condition	The USPSTF concludes that the current evidence is insufficient to assess the balance of benefits and harms of performing screening pelvic examinations in asymptomatic women for the early detection and treatment of a range of gynecologic conditions.	I	Examinations may be indicated for diagnostic considerations in symptomatic survivor patients. This measure refers to screening in asymptomatic patients.

APPENDIX. Sample United States Preventive Services Task Force (USPSTF) screening recommendations with special considerations for patients with a history of being trafficked (*continued*)

ISSUE AREA	POPULATION	RECOMMENDATION	GRADE	CONSIDERATIONS IN HUMAN TRAFFICKING
Hepatitis C: screening	Adults at high risk	The USPSTF recommends screening for hepatitis C virus (HCV) infection in persons at high risk for infection. The USPSTF also recommends offering one-time screening for HCV infection to adults born between 1945 and 1965.	B	Survivors of human trafficking should be considered high risk given their living and working conditions, including isolation, deprivation, violence, and exploitation.
Latent tuberculosis infection: screening	Asymptomatic adults at increased risk for infection	The USPSTF recommends screening for latent tuberculosis infection in populations at increased risk.	B	Survivors of human trafficking should be considered high risk given the living and working conditions, including overcrowding, exposure to high-risk populations, isolation, deprivation, violence, and exploitation.

APPENDIX. Sample United States Preventive Services Task Force (USPSTF) screening recommendations with special considerations for patients with a history of being trafficked (*continued*)

ISSUE AREA	POPULATION	RECOMMENDATION	GRADE	CONSIDERATIONS IN HUMAN TRAFFICKING
Lung cancer: screening	Adults ages 55–80 years, with a history of smoking	The USPSTF recommends annual screening for lung cancer with low-dose computed tomography in adults ages 55–80 years who have a 30 pack-year smoking history and currently smoke or have quit within the past 15 years. Screening should be discontinued once a person has not smoked for 15 years or develops a health problem that substantially limits life expectancy or the ability or willingness to have curative lung surgery.	B	Smoking may be a maladaptive coping mechanism in patients who have experienced trauma; it is essential to assess smoking history and risk for lung cancer and offer screening to affected survivor patients.

APPENDIX. Sample United States Preventive Services Task Force (USPSTF) screening recommendations with special considerations for patients with a history of being trafficked (*continued*)

ISSUE AREA	POPULATION	RECOMMENDATION	GRADE	CONSIDERATIONS IN HUMAN TRAFFICKING
Tobacco smoking cessation in adults, including pregnant women: behavioral interventions	Adults who are not pregnant	The USPSTF recommends that clinicians ask all adults about tobacco use, advise them to stop using tobacco, and provide behavioral interventions and U.S. FDA–approved pharmacotherapy for cessation to adults who use tobacco.	A	Smoking may be a maladaptive coping mechanism in patients who have experienced trauma; it is essential to discuss smoking cessation in affected survivor patients.
	Pregnant women	The USPSTF recommends that clinicians ask all pregnant women about tobacco use, advise them to stop using tobacco, and provide behavioral interventions for cessation to pregnant women who use tobacco.	A	Smoking may be a maladaptive coping mechanism in patients who have experienced trauma; it is essential to discuss smoking cessation in affected survivor patients.

APPENDIX. Sample United States Preventive Services Task Force (USPSTF) screening recommendations with special considerations for patients with a history of being trafficked (*continued*)

ISSUE AREA	POPULATION	RECOMMENDATION	GRADE	CONSIDERATIONS IN HUMAN TRAFFICKING
Depression in children and adolescents: screening	Adolescents ages 12–18 years	The USPSTF recommends screening for major depressive disorder (MDD) in adolescents ages 12–18 years. Screening should be implemented with adequate systems in place to ensure accurate diagnosis, effective treatment, and appropriate follow-up.	B	Labor and sex trafficking of children can have severe mental health effects, and screening should be conducted.
	Children age 11 years or younger	The USPSTF concludes that the current evidence is insufficient to assess the balance of benefits and harms of screening for MDD in children age 11 years or younger.	I	If there is a history of trafficking, then screening might be appropriate.

APPENDIX. Sample United States Preventive Services Task Force (USPSTF) screening recommendations with special considerations for patients with a history of being trafficked (*continued*)

ISSUE AREA	POPULATION	RECOMMENDATION	GRADE	CONSIDERATIONS IN HUMAN TRAFFICKING
Cervical cancer: screening	Women ages 21–65 years	The USPSTF recommends screening for cervical cancer every 3 years with cervical cytology alone in women ages 21–29 years. For women ages 30–65 years, the USPSTF recommends screening every 3 years with cervical cytology alone, every 5 years with high-risk human papillomavirus (hrHPV) testing alone, or every 5 years with hrHPV testing in combination with cytology (cotesting).	A	HPV exposure and risk of cervical cancer may be increased in sex trafficked and labor-trafficked patients, given lack of agency and control.
	Women older than 65 years	The USPSTF recommends against screening for cervical cancer in women older than 65 years who have had adequate prior screening and are not otherwise at high risk for cervical cancer.	D	It is important to assess possible history of exploitation, violence, and trafficking and to ensure that adequate prior screening occurred before ending screening in any patient over 65 years.

APPENDIX. Sample United States Preventive Services Task Force (USPSTF) screening recommendations with special considerations for patients with a history of being trafficked (*continued*)

ISSUE AREA	POPULATION	RECOMMENDATION	GRADE	CONSIDERATIONS IN HUMAN TRAFFICKING
Cervical cancer: screening (*continued*)	Women younger than 21 years	The USPSTF recommends against screening for cervical cancer in women younger than 21 years.	D	There is no evidence for screening in youth under 21 years; however, there may be indications for diagnostic examinations and testing if clinically indicated.
	Women who have had a hysterectomy	The USPSTF recommends against screening for cervical cancer in women who have had a hysterectomy with removal of the cervix and do not have a history of a high-grade precancerous lesion (i.e., cervical intraepithelial neoplasia [CIN] grade 2 or 3) or cervical cancer.	D	Women who have been trafficked may not know or have access to their medical history for procedures done while being trafficked. It is important to consider the history for accuracy before deciding to stop screening.

APPENDIX. Sample United States Preventive Services Task Force (USPSTF) screening recommendations with special considerations for patients with a history of being trafficked (*continued*)

ISSUE AREA	POPULATION	RECOMMENDATION	GRADE	CONSIDERATIONS IN HUMAN TRAFFICKING
Chlamydia and gonorrhea: screening	Sexually active women	The USPSTF recommends screening for chlamydia and gonorrhea in sexually active women age 24 years and younger and in older women who are at increased risk for infection.	B	All female patients who have been labor or sex trafficked, regardless of age, should be considered at increased risk for infection and should be screened because of lack of agency and control while being trafficked.
	Sexually active men	The USPSTF concludes that the current evidence is insufficient to assess the balance of benefits and harms of screening for chlamydia and gonorrhea in men.	I	Although there is inconclusive evidence to recommend for or against screening, it is important to consider that men who are trafficked lack agency and are subject to violence, abuse, and exploitation, including sexual violence. In discussion and consultation with the patient, the patient may decide to be screened for this reason alone.

APPENDIX. Sample United States Preventive Services Task Force (USPSTF) screening recommendations with special considerations for patients with a history of being trafficked (*continued*)

ISSUE AREA	POPULATION	RECOMMENDATION	GRADE	CONSIDERATIONS IN HUMAN TRAFFICKING
Hepatitis B virus infection: screening	Persons at high risk for infection	The USPSTF recommends screening for hepatitis B virus infection in persons at high risk for infection.	B	All patients who have been labor or sex trafficked should be considered at increased risk for infection and should be screened because of lack of agency and control while being trafficked, as well as the living and working conditions of deprivation, social restrictions, overcrowding, and possible dangerous/degrading/dirty labor conditions.
Intimate partner violence: screening	Women of reproductive age	The USPSTF recommends that clinicians screen for intimate partner violence in women of reproductive age and provide or refer women who screen positive to ongoing support services.	B	Human trafficking is inherently exploitative and violent. The clinician may want to assess for other forms of violence as well as intimate partner violence.

APPENDIX. Sample United States Preventive Services Task Force (USPSTF) screening recommendations with special considerations for patients with a history of being trafficked (*continued*)

ISSUE AREA	POPULATION	RECOMMENDATION	GRADE	CONSIDERATIONS IN HUMAN TRAFFICKING
Syphilis infection in nonpregnant adults and adolescents: screening	Asymptomatic, nonpregnant adults and adolescents who are at increased risk for syphilis infection	The USPSTF recommends screening for syphilis infection in persons who are at increased risk for infection.	A	All patients with a history of being trafficked should be screened for syphilis.
Unhealthy alcohol use in adolescents and adults: screening and behavioral counseling interventions	Adults 18 years or older, including pregnant women	The USPSTF recommends screening for unhealthy alcohol use in primary care settings in adults 18 years or older, including pregnant women, and providing persons engaged in risky or hazardous drinking with brief behavioral counseling interventions to reduce unhealthy alcohol use.	B	Given the possibility of trauma, and coercive use of substances, maladaptive coping behaviors, like unhealthy alcohol use, should be screened for in patients who have been trafficked.

APPENDIX. Sample United States Preventive Services Task Force (USPSTF) screening recommendations with special considerations for patients with a history of being trafficked (*continued*)

ISSUE AREA	POPULATION	RECOMMENDATION	GRADE	CONSIDERATIONS IN HUMAN TRAFFICKING
HIV infection: screening	Adolescents and adults ages 15–65 years	The USPSTF recommends that clinicians screen for HIV infection in adolescents and adults ages 15–65 years. Younger adolescents and older adults who are at increased risk should also be screened.	A	Just like any other patient in primary care, patients who have been trafficked should be screened for HIV.
	Pregnant women	The USPSTF recommends that clinicians screen all pregnant women for HIV, including those who present in labor who are untested and whose HIV status is unknown.	A	Just like any other patient in primary care, pregnant patients who have been trafficked should be screened for HIV.

For full recommendations, please visit www.uspreventiveservicestaskforce.org/Page/Name/recommendations.

CHAPTER 8

Responding to Trafficked Persons in Health Care Settings

PATIENT-CENTERED, SURVIVOR-CENTERED CARE

Susie B. Baldwin, M.D., M.P.H., FACPM

Holly Austin Gibbs, B.A.

Jordan Greenbaum, M.D.

Cathy L. Miller, R.N., Ph.D.

> The most disturbing thing was that they just did not know what to do with me.
>
> —*Survivor (Miller et al. 2016)*

A 16-year-old Guatemalan male was picked up by law enforcement after they received an anonymous tip about labor trafficking at a construction site. He and 12 others were identified as potential trafficking survivors. On the scene, a law enforcement officer noticed a dirty, poorly healing arm injury, so he brought the youth to the emergency department. When the health care provider attempted to obtain a medical history (using an interpreter), she found the patient withdrawn, angry, and reluctant to speak. He did not make eye contact and gave one-word answers. He did not provide details about how he sustained the injury and refused examination.

When developing policies and procedures for responding to patients who may be trafficked, it is essential to utilize a patient-centered framework, in which we respect and value patients' perspectives. *NEJM Catalyst* notes that "in patient-centered care, an individual's specific health needs and desired health outcomes are the driving force behind all health care decisions and quality measurements.

Patients are partners with their health care providers, and providers treat patients not only from a clinical perspective, but also from an emotional, mental, spiritual, social, and financial perspective" (NEJM Catalyst 2017; see also Institute of Medicine 2001).

The trauma inherent to both sex and labor trafficking impacts all these perspectives and affects how survivors engage with service providers and authority figures, including doctors, nurses, social workers, and counselors. To effectively assist patients who have been trafficked, we must appreciate the complexities of human trafficking and our appropriate role in addressing it. Although we must be prepared to help survivors connect with resources or exit their exploitive situation when they are ready and willing to do so, we also need to understand that health care providers seldom find opportunities to "rescue" patients from their situation. However, every encounter with a vulnerable patient or a patient in whom we suspect exploitation or trafficking is an opportunity to educate and empower that person, moving them along a pathway to self-determination and safety.

Two fundamental aspects of a patient-centered, survivor-centered approach for people who have survived violence are 1) trauma-informed service delivery and 2) utilization of a universal education, nondisclosure approach to assessment (Miller et al. 2011). In this chapter, we discuss the application of these frameworks in the context of human trafficking.

IMPORTANCE OF A TRAUMA-INFORMED APPROACH

Trauma and traumatic stress are inherent to human trafficking. Terms such as *force*, *fraud*, *coercion*, and *exploitation* imply experiences of trauma, betrayal, uncertainty, and powerlessness. To understand a trafficked person's beliefs, attitudes, and behaviors, a health care professional must appreciate the impact of the (frequently) complex trauma sustained by that individual before, during, and after a period of exploitation. A trauma-informed approach to patient or client interaction implies that the health care professional has an understanding of trauma and its impact, can recognize signs/symptoms of traumatic stress, and is committed to responding in a nonjudgmental, empathic, and respectful manner that minimizes retraumatization and maximizes patient or client empowerment (Substance Abuse and Mental Health Services Administration 2014). Trauma-informed care embodies six principles:

1. Safety (both physical and psychological)
2. Trustworthiness and transparency in actions
3. Collaboration and mutuality (e.g., minimization of the power differential and facilitation of shared decision-making)
4. Empowerment, voice, and choice (e.g., focus on resiliency, actively seeking to empower the patient or client and encourage self-advocacy)
5. Peer support (e.g., shared experiences, emphasis on building trust and hope between peers)
6. Acknowledgment of cultural, historical and gender issues (e.g., recognition of, respect for, and sensitivity to differences in culture, race/ethnicity, religion, age, gender, sexual orientation, and nationality and efforts to incorporate the healing value of the patient's or client's culture and religion into treatment strategies)

A trauma-informed organization incorporates these principles into policies, procedures, and everyday interactions between staff and patients/clients.

Qualitative studies documenting the survivor perspective on health, mental health, and other services consistently demonstrate a need and desire for trauma-informed care. Participants have reported experiences of blaming, stigmatization, and insensitivity by professionals (Baldwin et al. 2011; Ijadi-Maghsoodi et al. 2018; Ravi et al. 2017).

> I went to the ER and it was the most awkward thing ever…they treated it more like—as like a rape victim…. And then, the doctor was just like, "So you were prostituting?" And I was like, "No." I was like "Well, I mean, yes" …" And, I didn't want to go to a doctor ever again, like, for months after that…there was like no sensitivity…. (survivor quote from Rajaram and Tidball 2018, p. 193)

Survivor recommendations for improving patient and client care include adopting a nonjudgmental, nonbiased, empathic approach, with a focus on psychological safety, client empowerment and choice, and a commitment to confidentiality (Corbett 2018; Ijadi-Maghsoodi et al. 2018; Rajaram and Tidball 2018). In short, survivors are calling for trauma-informed care.

IMPORTANCE OF UNIVERSAL EDUCATION

Many variables contribute to a health care professional's ability, or inability, to identify trafficked persons in health care settings. The barriers to identification may be system related, professional, or patient related, resulting in a lack of recognition of the patient as a trafficked person (Miller et al. 2016). The lack of identification of trafficked persons in health care settings results in missed opportunities for the health care professional to provide appropriate treatment, assistance, referral, and patient education.

Peer-reviewed and gray literature has demonstrated that health care professionals commonly do not recognize trafficked persons who present for health care services and that survivors are not likely to recognize or disclose their victimization (Baldwin et al. 2011; Lumpkin and Taboada 2017; Lederer and Wetzel 2014; Rajaram and Tidball 2018). This gap necessitates a shift in the way we assess for human trafficking victimization. We call for a universal education approach that involves a health care professional providing health education and anticipatory guidance to all patients (Futures Without Violence 2019; Greenbaum et al. 2015; Miller et al. 2011).

Universal education is the concept of health care providers giving anticipatory guidance to all patients regardless of their chief complaint, gender, or sexual orientation, but such education may be more important for those most at risk for victimization (Miller et al. 2015). While understanding that exploitation and trafficking come in many forms and impact populations across all demographic, social, and economic lines, it is important to be aware that groups at increased risk include runaway youth and people experiencing homelessness, youth involved in juvenile justice or child welfare systems, immigrants working in the low-wage service economy, people with limited English proficiency, people with disabilities, and people who identify as lesbian, gay, bisexual, transgender, or otherwise queer (LGBTQ).

In the context of patient assessment for human trafficking and other forms of interpersonal violence, such as intimate partner violence and sexual assault, universal education teaches patients that violence and coercion are related to their well-being, providing patients the space to discuss personal and difficult issues with their clinician. Shifting the screening and treatment paradigm to include a universal education approach serves two primary purposes: to align with 1) the provision of trauma-informed care and survivor/patient–centered care to empower the patient with education and choices, and 2) a public health approach to advance primary, secondary, and tertiary prevention (Miller et al. 2011) rather than simply screening and treating patients for their immediate problems.

Trauma-informed care requires that health care professionals and organizations integrate a universal delivery of compassionate, respectful survivor/patient–centered care into their operations. The proactive approach to empowering all patients with education, anticipatory guidance, and choices transcends the onetime encounter, providing patients with information and resources at the time of the visit and longitudinally and to share with family and friends. This preventive approach holds the promise of making hospitals, clinics, and doctors' offices more welcoming to trafficking survivors and could ultimately improve outcomes for survivors.

THE PEARR TOOL

In partnership with HEAL Trafficking and Pacific Survivor Center, Dignity Health (2018), a member of CommonSpirit Health, developed the PEARR Tool to help guide social workers, nurses, physicians, and other professionals on how to provide assistance in a trauma-informed manner. PEARR is an acronym for the following steps: **P**rovide privacy, **E**ducate, **A**sk, **R**espect, and **R**espond.

The PEARR Tool is based on a universal education model, which has been popularized by Futures Without Violence as part of their CUES Intervention (Futures Without Violence 2019). In this CUES Intervention model, health professionals are encouraged to use safety cards to talk with all patients about healthy and unhealthy relationships and the health effects of violence. Disclosure is not the goal; however, disclosures will occur. If a patient discloses an unhealthy relationship, then the health professional is encouraged to discuss a patient-centered care plan with the patient, which includes making a warm referral (i.e., a personal introduction) to a service provider. After caring for numerous patients who have exhibited indicators of human trafficking and other forms of violence, and after debriefing with staff on many of these cases, Dignity Health has determined that universal education may be key in prevention and intervention for many forms of abuse, neglect, and violence, including human trafficking.

Dignity Health, HEAL Trafficking, and Pacific Survivor Center recommend providing universal education about various forms of abuse, neglect, and violence in all health care settings, particularly in nonacute care settings that offer longitudinal care and services. For urgent and emergency care settings, a universal education approach may be most appropriate and effective when a patient presents with risk factors or indicators of victimization. In this case, the PEARR Tool offers guidance to health care professionals about how to provide education and assistance in a trauma-informed manner.

The first step of the PEARR Tool involves providing a patient with a safe and private setting, ideally a private room with closed doors. If a companion refuses to be separated from a patient, even briefly, then this may be an indicator of abuse, neglect, or violence. Consider strategies to separate the patient from the companion in a non-threatening manner. For example, state the requirement for a private exam or a need for the patient to accompany you alone for a radiology or urine test, or request the companion's assistance with completing registration forms in the lobby.

If a companion still refuses to be separated from a patient and you suspect abuse, neglect, or violence may be a concern, then it *may not* be safe to insist on separation. As described by the Office for Victims of Crime, a "victim-centered approach" means the person's wishes, safety, and well-being are prioritized in all matters and procedures. In this case, it may not be safe to separate the patient and companion. Instead, continue health services as normal but notify appropriate staff (e.g., a security officer) about any safety concerns and concerns of abuse, neglect, or violence as required or permitted by law or regulation (Office for Victims of Crime 2019).

If you are able to speak with the patient alone, then explain any limits to confidentiality with the patient before beginning a sensitive discussion about abuse, neglect, or violence. Limits to confidentiality include your legal requirements to report suspicions of abuse, neglect, or violence to external agencies according to law or regulation. To explain limits of confidentiality, you must fully understand your mandated reporting requirements as outlined by federal, state, and/or local law and regulation.

The next step is to educate the patient about abuse, neglect, or violence in a nonjudgmental and normalized manner. For example, you may, as in the PEARR tool, begin a conversation as follows: "I educate all of my patients about [fill in the blank] because violence is so common in our society, and violence can have a big impact on our health, safety, and well-being. Let's review some information together" (Dignity Health 2018). Beginning a conversation with a patient in this way can reduce tension between the health care professional and the patient, and it can encourage open communication.

Determining which types of abuse, neglect, or violence are discussed should be based on the health care setting and on the presence of any risk factors or indicators of victimization. To learn more about risk factors and indicators associated with child abuse or neglect, see the website of the Child Welfare Information Gateway (www.child-welfare.gov). For risk factors and indicators associated with the abuse or neglect of vulnerable adults (e.g., elder and dependent adults), see the National Adult Protective Services Association's website (www.napsa-now.org) and Centers for Disease Control and Prevention website (Centers for Disease Control and Prevention 2019).

Risk factors and indicators associated with domestic violence and intimate partner violence are provided by the National Domestic Violence Hotline (www.thehotline.org) and the CDC (Centers for Disease Control and Prevention 2007). For risk factors and indicators associated with sexual violence, see the Rape, Abuse and Incest National Network (www.rainn.org) and the CDC (Centers for Disease Control and Prevention 2007). For risk factors and indicators associated with labor and sex trafficking, see the National Human Trafficking Hotline's resource "What to Look for in a Health Care Setting" (National Human Trafficking Hotline 2016).

Use of a brochure or safety card is recommended when reviewing information about abuse, neglect, or violence with a patient. Ideally, this brochure or safety card will include information about resources (e.g., national hotlines). For example, the National Runaway Safeline offers free downloadable brochures along with wallet cards in English and Spanish (www.1800runaway.org/free-promotional-materials). Their general brochure describes an overview of services available to runaway, homeless, and at-risk youth.

Futures Without Violence also offers numerous free resources for patients in various languages, including safety cards that provide information about health and safety issues related to domestic violence/intimate partner violence. Many of these safety cards are designed for specific populations (e.g., American Indians/Alaska Natives, Hawaiians, and persons who identify as LGBTQ or gender nonconforming.

In partnership with the National Survivor Network (nationalsurvivornetwork.org) and Eleven Inc., Dignity Health is working to develop a brochure that will include information about human trafficking for patients who may be survivors. Until this brochure is completed, the following resources are available:

- The Federal Bureau of Investigation (2019) offers a brochure, *Help for Victims of Trafficking in Persons*—available in English, Spanish, Chinese, Japanese, Korean, and Tagalog.

- The Office on Trafficking in Persons, an office of the Administration for Children and Families, offers the following brochures to health care and related professionals:

  - *Human Trafficking: Information for Health Care Providers* (Administration for Children and Families 2019a)—available in English and Spanish
  - *FACT SHEET: Human Trafficking*—available in English (Administration for Children and Families 2017)
  - *Look Beneath the Surface: Child Exploitation Brochure*—available in English, Indonesian, Korean, Spanish, Thai, and Vietnamese (Administration for Children and Families 2019b)
  - *Look Beneath the Surface: Health Care Brochure*—available in English and Spanish (Administration for Children and Families 2019c)
  - *Look Beneath the Surface: Social Services Brochure*—available in English, Spanish, Chinese, Korean, Thai, Vietnamese, and Indonesian (Administration for Children and Families 2019d)

In addition Homeland Security's Blue Campaign (www.dhs.gov/blue-campaign) offers numerous resources for building awareness about human trafficking in the community. Their online document library includes information sheets, pamphlets, and cards in various languages.

After reviewing information about abuse, neglect, or violence, allow time for open discussion with the patient, especially if the patient is exhibiting risk factors or indicators of victimization. For example, according to the PEARR Tool (Dignity Health 2018), you may say, "Is there anything you'd like to share with me?" or "Do you feel like anyone is hurting your health, safety, or well-being?" If a patient is open to answering questions, then consider use of an evidence-based tool to screen the patient for abuse, neglect, or violence.

For example, the U.S. Preventive Services Task Force recommends that clinicians screen all women of childbearing age for domestic violence and intimate partner violence (recommendation Grade B; U.S. Preventive Services Task Force et al. 2018). The U.S. Preventive Services Task Force also lists several screening tools available for use in the health care setting, including the Hurt, Insult, Threaten, and Scream Tool (HITS; Bardwell et al. 1999.; Sherin et al. 1998). HITS is also validated for use with men (Shakil et al. 2005). For additional information about HITS and other screening and assessment tools, see *Intimate Partner Violence and Sexual Vi-*

olence Victimization Assessment Instruments for Use in Healthcare Settings, a publication from the CDC (Centers for Disease Control and Prevention 2007).

For information about child abuse or neglect screening tools, see the Child Welfare Information Gateway (www.childwelfare.gov). For information about tools that screen for elder abuse, see *Elder Abuse Screening Tools for Healthcare Professionals*, a publication from the National Center on Elder Abuse (2016). For information about tools available to screen patients for labor or sex trafficking victimization, see the resources provided by HEAL Trafficking (https://healtrafficking.org).

If a patient is exhibiting indicators of victimization, then ask the patient directly about safety concerns. For example, according to the PEARR Tool (Dignity Health 2018), you may say, "I've noticed [insert risk factor/indicator], and I'm concerned for your health, safety, and well-being. You don't have to share details with me, but I'd like to connect you with someone who may be able to help you. Would you like to speak with [insert victim advocate/service provider]? If not, and you change your mind, you can let me know anytime. I'm here to help."

The final step is *to respect and respond* accordingly. If the patient denies victimization or declines assistance, then respect the patient's wishes. This may be the most difficult step for a health care professional to take; however, this respect for the patient's decisions is key to providing a victim-centered and trauma-informed approach. Education about trauma, including the prevalence and widespread impact of trauma and the potential signs and symptoms of trauma in patients and others, can help a professional better understand a patient's wishes to protect an abuser or decline services.

If a patient denies victimization or declines assistance, and you still have concerns about abuse, neglect, or violence, then offer the patient information about resources that can assist in the event of an emergency (e.g., local service providers, national hotlines). Ideally, this information will be printed on a small card or other item that the patient can hide in their belongings. For example, the National Human Trafficking Hotline offers pocket cards in numerous languages. If the patient chooses to accept the card, they can hide it in a pocket or shoe.

Otherwise, if the patient accepts or requests assistance with accessing services, then provide the patient with a warm referral to a local victim advocate or service provider, according to the patient's wishes. It is imperative to identify *ahead of time* any local, state, or national resources, both public and private agencies, that can provide services and support to patients who may be victims and/or survivors of abuse, neglect, or violence. If local resources are limited, arrange a private setting for the patient to call a national hotline (e.g., the National Domestic Violence Hotline, 1-800-799-SAFE [7233], www.thehotline.org; National Sexual Assault Hotline, 1-800-656-HOPE [4673], www.rainn.org/about-national-sexual-assault-telephone-hotline; and National Human Trafficking Hotline, 1-888-373-7888, https://humantraffickinghotline.org).

Throughout the text of the PEARR Tool, a double asterisk (**) indicates points at which this sensitive conversation with a patient may come to an end, for example, if a patient's companion refuses to be separated from the patient. If you are unable to begin a private conversation with a patient—or once this private conversation ends— refer to the double asterisk at the bottom of the first page of the PEARR Tool, which provides additional steps: 1) report safety concerns to appropriate personnel (e.g., nurse supervisor, patient safety/security officer), 2) report risk factors or indicators as required or permitted by law/regulation, and 3) continue health services in a trauma-informed manner.

Whenever possible, a follow-up appointment should be scheduled in order to continue building rapport with the patient and to monitor the patient's health, safety, and well-being (to download a copy of the PEARR Tool, go to www.dignityhealth.org/hello-humankindness/human-trafficking/victim-centered-and-trauma-informed).

CONCLUSION

Trafficking and exploitation involve considerable trauma and distress to affected persons, often with deprivation and extensive abuse. To best serve trafficked persons, clinicians can adopt a trauma-informed, culturally sensitive, rights-based approach that suspends judgment and respects survivor autonomy. This strategy for patient care emphasizes an appreciation for the effects of trauma on a patient's beliefs, behaviors, and attitudes; an open demeanor; active listening; and conscientious attention to the need for privacy, safety, informed consent, and patient empowerment. We advocate an approach that includes the practice of universal education about violence to let patients know that experiences of coercion and abuse are harmful to their health, coupled with assessment and screening for abuse that do not exclusively aim for patient disclosure. Universal education about human trafficking, with an offer of local and national resources, may provide at-risk individuals critical information for future change.

Pearls and Pointers

- A trauma-informed, culturally sensitive, survivor-centered, rights-based approach to patient care maximizes the likelihood of building trust with a patient and making the health visit a positive experience.

- Persons who have been trafficked may not disclose their exploitation, trauma, and distress. Universal education about violence and health, with an offer of resources, can enable clinicians to help those in need without necessitating disclosure.

- The PEARR tool is a useful aid for providing services to traumatized individuals.

- To empower trafficking survivors and assist them on their journeys toward healing, clinicians must respect their decisions about their health and lives, even when we disagree. (With minor victims, many decisions lay in our hands, but we should allow autonomy whenever possible.)

- It is essential for health care providers to appreciate the impact of trauma on health and behavior; by doing so, we can greatly improve care for individual patients. However, care for patients who have experienced trafficking and other forms of violence can only be optimized within health care organizations that implement systemwide trauma-informed practices and policies.

REFERENCES

Administration for Children and Families: FACT SHEET: human trafficking. November 21, 2017. Available at: www.acf.hhs.gov/sites/default/files/otip/fact_sheet_human_trafficking_fy18.pdf. Accessed November 5, 2019.

Administration for Children and Families: Human trafficking: information for health care providers. 2019a. Available at: www.acf.hhs.gov/sites/default/files/otip/lbs_hc_brochure_eng.pdf. Accessed April 15, 2020.

Administration for Children and Families: Look Beneath the Surface: child exploitation brochure. 2019b. Available at: www.acf.hhs.gov/sites/default/files/orr/child_exploitation_brochure.pdf. Accessed April 15, 2020.

Administration for Children and Families: Look Beneath the Surface—health care brochure. 2019c. Available at: www.acf.hhs.gov/sites/default/files/endtrafficking/healthcare_brochure_nov2016.pdf. Accessed November 5, 2019.

Administration for Children and Families: Look Beneath the Surface: social services brochure. 2019d. Available at: www.acf.hhs.gov/sites/default/files/orr/look_beneath_the_surface_brochure_1_english.pdf. Accessed November April 15, 2020.

Baldwin S, Eisenman D, Sayles J, et al: Identification of human trafficking victims in health care settings. Health Human Rights 13(1):E36–E49, 2011 22772961

Bardwell J, Sherin K, Sinacore J, et al: Screening for domestic violence in family medicine. Journal of Advocate Health Care 1(1):5–7, 1999

Centers for Disease Control and Prevention: Intimate Partner Violence and Sexual Violence Victimization Assessment Instruments for Use in Healthcare Settings. National Center for Injury Prevention and Control, 2007. Available at: www.cdc.gov/violenceprevention/pdf/ipv/ipvandsvscreening.pdf. Accessed November 5, 2019.

Centers for Disease Control and Prevention: Elder abuse. May 28, 2019. Available at: www.cdc.gov/violenceprevention/elderabuse/index.html. Accessed November 5, 2019.

Corbett A: The voices of survivors: an exploration of the contributing factors that assisted with exiting from commercial sexual exploitation in childhood. Children and Youth Services Review 85:91–98, 2018

Dignity Health: PEARR Tool: trauma-informed approach to victim assistance in health care settings. 2018. Available at: www.dignityhealth.org//media/cm/media/documents/PDFs/PEARRToolm15NoField2019.ashx?la=en&hash=F14648F8505CF79BAA9B62B87B6C584802673D3A. Accessed November 5, 2019.

Federal Bureau of Investigation: Help for victims of trafficking in persons. 2019. Available at: www.fbi.gov/file-repository/help-for-victims-of-trafficking-brochure.pdf/view. Accessed November 5, 2019.

Futures Without Violence: IPV Health: Adopt the evidence-based CUES intervention to support survivors and prevent violence. 2019, Available at: http://ipvhealth.org/health-professionals/educate-providers. Accessed March 30, 2020.

Greenbaum J, Crawford-Jakubiak JE; Committee on Child Abuse and Neglect: Child sex trafficking and commercial sexual exploitation: health care needs of victims. Pediatrics 135(3):566–574, 2015 25713283

Ijadi-Maghsoodi R, Bath E, Cook M, et al: Commercially sexually exploited youths' health care experiences, barriers, and recommendations: a qualitative analysis. Child Abuse Negl 76:334–341, 2018 29195171

Institute of Medicine: Crossing the Quality Chasm: A New Health System for the 21st Century. Washington, DC, National Academy Press, 2001

Lederer L, Wetzel C: The health consequences of sex trafficking and their implications for identifying victims in healthcare facilities. Annals of Health Law 23:61–91, 2014

Lumpkin CL, Taboada A: Identification and referral for human trafficking survivors in health care settings: survey report. Coalition to Abolish Slavery and Human Trafficking, CastLA.org, Jan 13, 2017. Available at: www.castla.org/wp-content/themes/castla/assets/files/ Identification_and_Referral_in_Health_Care_Settings_survey_report_ 2017.pdf. Accessed March 22, 2020.

Miller CL, Duke G, Northam S: Child sex-trafficking recognition, intervention, and referral: An educational framework to the development of health care provider education programs. Journal of Human Trafficking 2(3):177–200, 2016

Miller E, Decker MR, McCauley HL, et al: A family planning clinic partner violence intervention to reduce risk associated with reproductive coercion. Contraception 83(3):274–280, 2011 21310291

Miller E, Goldstein S, McCauley HL, et al: A school health center intervention for abusive adolescent relationships: a cluster RCT. Pediatrics 135(1):76–85, 2015 25535265

National Center on Elder Abuse: Elder abuse screening tools for healthcare professionals. 2016. Available at: http://eldermistreatment.usc.edu/wp-content/uploads/2016/10/Elder-Abuse-Screening-Tools-for-Healthcare-Professionals.pdf. Accessed November 5, 2019.

National Human Trafficking Hotline: What to look for in a health care setting. February 2016. Available at: https://humantraffickinghotline.org/ resources/what-look-healthcare-setting. Accessed November 5, 2019.

NEJM Catalyst: What is patient-centered care? NEJM Catalyst Jan 1, 2016

Office for Victims of Crime: Human Trafficking Task Force e-guide: strengthening collaborative responses. 2019. Available at: www.ovcttac.gov/ taskforceguide/eguide/1-understanding-human-trafficking/13-victim-centered-approach/. Accessed November 5, 2019.

Rajaram SS, Tidball S: Survivors' voices—complex needs of sex trafficking survivors in the Midwest. Behav Med 44(3):189–198, 2018 29095121

Ravi A, Pfeiffer MR, Rosner Z, et al: Trafficking and trauma: insight and advice for the healthcare system from sex-trafficked women incarcerated on Rikers Island. Med Care 55(12):1017–1022, 2017 28945674

Shakil A, Donald S, Sinacore JM, et al: Validation of the HITS domestic violence screening tool with males. Fam Med 37(3):193–198, 2005 15739135

Sherin KM, Sinacore JM, Li XQ, et al: HITS: a short domestic violence screening tool for use in a family practice setting. Fam Med 30(7):508–512, 1998 9669164

Substance Abuse and Mental Health Services Administration: SAMHSA's concept of trauma and guidance for a trauma-informed approach. July 2014. Available at: https://store.samhsa.gov/system/files/sma14-4884.pdf. Accessed November 5, 2019.

U.S. Preventive Services Task Force, Curry SJ, Krist AH, et al: Screening for intimate partner violence, elder abuse, and abuse of vulnerable adults: US Preventive Services Task Force final recommendation statement. JAMA 320(16):1678–1687, 2018 30357305

Care Management of Trafficked Persons With Substance Use Disorders

Yasmine Omar, Ph.D.

Gabriela Austgen, M.D.

Nidal Moukaddam, M.D., Ph.D.

> You can sell a drug once, but you can sell the human body time and time again.
>
> *—Anonymous*

Rae was 14 when she left home. For the previous 2 years, she had spent as much time as possible with her aunt, her grandmother, and even a friend from school whose parents felt bad for her in desperate attempts to avoid her mother's home. But her family members and friends made it clear that although they loved her, they couldn't help her anymore. There are considerable expenses related to raising a teenager, and these families were struggling as it was.

But the environment of Rae's home was toxic: her mother could not protect her from her stepfather and sought refuge in painkillers and vodka. Her stepfather, although fully providing financially for the family, had been emotionally abusive for as long as she could remember. One particularly painful memory she had was of him threatening to shoot her dog should she stand up to him again.

With all this mental baggage, Rae was not doing well at school. She had smoked cannabis, but she had also promised herself never to become her mother, who was dependent on her stepfather and unable to leave her environment because of addiction.

Rae started staying with a group of older teenagers whose parents were never home. An older "cousin" would sometimes visit. He was nice to her. He asked questions and seemed to listen to her story. And one fateful day, when she was upset about her mother, he gave her a white powder to try, saying, "Here, it will make you feel better."

What ensued was a nightmarish period of 2 years during which Rae became increasingly addicted to the substance. She started with snorting. She quickly graduated to intravenous drug use after the same older individual injected her for the first time. She tried to leave, but when she did, she experienced intense humiliation. All the secrets she had divulged were turned against her. The older teens knew she had nowhere to go. They also knew that if she failed to keep up the required charade, her mother would be in trouble for truancy, as Rae was still a minor. She did not feel she could trust the school counselor or her family.

As the addiction cycle deepened and the demands placed on her increased, she was forced to steal from stores and then attempt to return the stolen items for refunds. She was also forced to apply for food stamps and other benefits fraudulently. After an escape attempt, she was raped. Even in the absence of threats, she was afraid to leave, as she feared the intensity of her drug withdrawal symptoms.

Escape came in the form of an overdose that needed medical intervention. The medical team did not believe her story and asked to interview her alone. This was the first time she had a chance to disclose the circumstances of her plight. She was scared, but said enough to trigger an admission, followed by a report to child protective services. From this point forward, her life would begin changing for the better.

PREVALENCE OF SUBSTANCE USE DISORDERS IN TRAFFICKED PERSONS

Among other mental health problems faced by trafficked persons, substance use disorders (SUDs) are extremely common. For purposes of this chapter, we define *substance use disorder* as a problematic pattern of use of an intoxicating substance, leading to clinically significant impairment or distress as outlined by DSM-5 (American Psychiatric Association 2013). Substance use disorders have been found to be highly comorbid with other trauma-related disorders, and throughout this chapter, we will discuss how screening for SUDs should be a routine part of assessment and treatment in this vulnerable population (Gerassi 2018). The high prevalence of SUDs in survivors of human trafficking argues for a multidisciplinary, trauma-informed approach to treatment. However, studies in this area remain scarce, and, as explained in this chapter, some of the general principles of addiction treatment may require adjustment to fit the needs of trafficked patients. The prevalence of SUDs in trafficked populations is high for various reasons. An interplay exists between trafficking and SUDs, and this can play a role in initiation, maintenance, and escalation of SUDs (Figure 9–1).

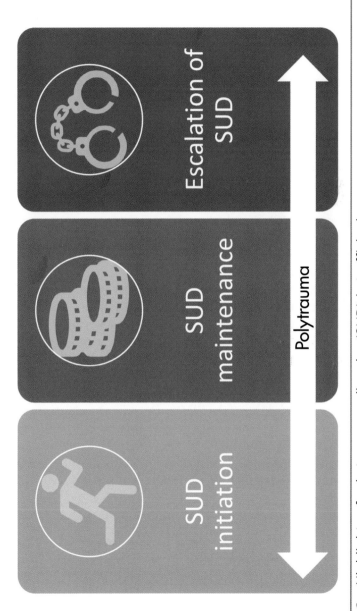

FIGURE 9–1. Highlights of substance use disorder (SUD) in trafficked persons.

SUDs are highly prevalent in trafficked persons, and escalating drug use, high levels of coercion, and mental health sequelae contribute to polytrauma.

Traffickers sometimes provide substances to those being trafficked as a way of keeping them debilitated and more easily trapped (Cook et al. 2018). In one survey of female trafficked persons, "more than a quarter (27.9%) said that forced substance use was a part of their trafficking experience. More than a quarter of victims reported injected drugs and overdoses" (Lederer and Wetzel 2014, p. 76). Conversely, trafficked persons may initiate substance use as a coping tool during and after their trafficking experience (Reid and Piquero 2014), similar to other survivors of traumatic experiences who suffer from posttraumatic stress.

Illicit drug use is itself considered a risk factor for human trafficking, even without preexisting trauma, because victims may place themselves in risky situations to secure their drugs and may deal with less than trustworthy individuals who will ask for illicit acts in exchange for drugs, resulting in what is now recognized as human trafficking (Le et al. 2018). Simply stated, trafficked persons engage in high-risk behavior, including commercial sexual activity, to financially support continued drug use (Varma et al. 2015). Farley et al. (2004) make the case that this is largely a myth and that in the majority of cases, substance use increases "to the point of addiction" after entry into prostitution, highlighting the role of human trafficking in maintenance and escalation of SUDs. This impression is based on interviews of individuals engaged in prostitution in nine countries, and the authors note that the severity of SUDs, as well as the severity of mental symptoms, was related to the extent of trauma incurred by the victims. Thus, engaging in high-risk behaviors is not enough initially to fuel the trafficking or the SUD cycle; it is when both combine and become routine that the victim is truly prisoner of the lifestyle.

Although there are few studies on this topic, the available literature consistently shows a high prevalence of SUDs in trafficked persons. Five studies (listed in Table 9–1) reported prevalence ranging from 46.9% to 92%.

The studies listed in Table 9–1 are limited in the demographics of groups surveyed, particularly with regard to age and sex. The vast majority of individuals included in all studies are women, and four of five focus on youth under the age of 18 years. Additionally, the cited populations exclude trafficked persons who do not come to the attention of medical providers or the criminal justice system. Furthermore, the prevalence data are not fine-grained enough to distinguish among types of trafficking, including sexual/labor exploitation or domestic servitude, and a corresponding SUD prevalence. It would be logical to assume that earlier exploitation and polytrauma

TABLE 9–1. Prevalence of substance use disorders (SUDs) in trafficked patients

STUDY	DEMOGRAPHIC	SAMPLE SIZE	PREVALENCE OF SUDS
Cook et al. 2018	Female youth participating in a specialty trafficking court program in Los Angeles, California; mean age 16 years	184	88%
Moore et al. 2017	Youth (under the age of 18 years; mean age 15.4 years) who disclosed their involvement in DMST to a medical provider; mostly female	25	92%
Landers et al. 2017	Youth ages 9–18 years living in Miami-Dade County, Florida, in the child welfare dependency system and identified as having serious mental or behavioral health problems; mean age 16.1 years and mostly female	87	46.9%
Goldberg et al. 2017	Youth under the age of 18 years referred for DMST at a Rhode Island hospital; mean age 15.5 years and mostly female	41	88%
Lederer and Wetzel 2014	Female sex trafficking survivors in the United States (adolescents and adults)	107	84%

Note. Various studies report different numbers. DMST=domestic minor sex trafficking.

would be associated with higher SUD rates and more severe SUD presentations, but conclusive comparative surveys are lacking.

A variety of substances (both legal and illegal) are used by survivors of human trafficking (Lederer and Wetzel 2014). The most common substances are alcohol, marijuana, and cocaine according to Lederer and Wetzel (use reported by over 50% of the survivors), as opposed to heroin, which was used by 22.3%. However, opioid use seems to have a particular link with human trafficking in the United States, a fact that is becoming more apparent as more is learned about the current opioid crisis (Stoklosa 2016). A recent example of this association that garnered national attention involved a Massachusetts sex trafficker who was sentenced to 17 years in prison for controlling women by exploiting their opioid addictions. According to a press release issued by the U.S. Department of Justice in 2018, "The defendant controlled the victims by supplying them with just enough heroin to avoid opiate withdrawal, which involves severe pain and physical sickness, and then threatening to cut off their supply and cause them to suffer withdrawal if they refused to engage in commercial sex" (U.S. Department of Justice 2018). One expert in human trafficking, an emergency department physician, observed that more than 50% of trafficked persons who presented to her emergency department were addicted to opioids (Stoklosa 2016). Stoklosa and colleagues (2017) concluded in another article that because of the strong link, opioid use itself may be an indication to screen for trafficking.

SUBSTANCE USE DISORDER DIAGNOSTIC CONSIDERATIONS AMONG TRAFFICKED PERSONS

There are several important factors to consider before engaging victims and trafficked persons in substance use treatment. Shandro and colleagues (2016) noted that because of their heterogeneity of experiences and needs, trafficked persons would benefit from a multidisciplinary approach to support. This includes establishing safe shelter, health care access, legal help, and treatment for SUDs.

Timing of treatment is critical, however, because trafficked persons may continue to abuse substances even after they are no longer trafficked (Macy and Johns 2011) as a way to cope with their trafficking experiences (Clawson et al. 2009; Raymond and Hughes 2001). It is unsurprising that substance use treatment in particular may be underutilized by this population (Caliber 2007; Clawson and Dutch 2008).

ASSESSMENT AND SCREENING

Because of this population's unique complexity, assessment of SUDs requires a thorough understanding of other hardships experienced by trafficked persons. A primary manifesting concern may not be substance use at all; a meta-analysis by Oram et al. (2016) identified difficulties with memory as well as somatic symptoms and pain (e.g., headache, back pain, stomach pain) to be the most common physical symptoms that trafficked persons report. The most frequent psychological difficulty faced by this population may be trauma related. Yakushko (2009) found that human trafficking survivors frequently display symptoms of having survived torture, including "psychosomatic reactions, psychological reactions, psychoactive substance abuse and dependence, social reactions, and psychophysical consequences of STDs or injuries" (p. 161). Because of the multiple or prolonged traumatic experiences of human trafficking, victims may exhibit signs of complex trauma, putting them at a higher risk of emotional dysregulation, psychological disorders, and substance use. These reports suggest that assessment of SUDs may be more effective if conducted within the context of a thorough assessment for a trafficked individual.

It is worth noting that assessment of SUDs in the general population may reduce vulnerability to human trafficking. Gibbons and Stoklosa (2016) discuss the case of an individual with a significant history of abuse as a child who had an SUD for multiple years as an adult. She attempted treatment multiple times and during a relapse fell into a sex-trafficking situation. This example highlights the importance of recognizing that human trafficking is not always the cause of an SUD; it may become an exacerbating consequence of the substance use. When patients are being assessed for SUDs, it is critical to recognize the comorbidity between trauma and substance use, regardless of the direction of causation.

TREATMENT CONSIDERATIONS

As noted earlier in this chapter, timing of treatment for SUDs is a delicate matter because of survivors' immediate needs for stability, safety, emergency medical care, and legal advocacy (Macy and Johns 2011). In fact, evidence suggests that providing secure housing and case management to an individual enrolling in substance use treatment increases drug abstinence rates and reduces relapse rates. In addition, Aron et al. (2006) found that trafficked persons frequently indicated that they wish to receive counseling treatment, specifically after they obtained a sense of safety and normalcy. Once these needs have been addressed, trafficked persons may be ready to, as Macy and Johns (2011) note, recover from the trauma of their experience and benefit from services addressing "a) physical health, b) mental health, c) substance abuse problems, d) safety, e) transitional housing, f) immigration, g) legal issues, and h) language needs" (p. 95). Macy and Johns (2011) also assert that the consensus in reviewed literature is that substance use treatment is a critical aspect of comprehensive services for trafficked persons.

Because of the high comorbidity between symptoms of trauma and substance use in this population, combined treatments for both trauma and SUDs are more effective than fragmented treatments. Some studies have found that, when tailored for substance use treatment, cognitive interventions such as cognitive processing therapy and its adapted version that eliminates developing a written trauma account, cognitive-only cognitive processing therapy, may be effective in reducing both trauma and substance use symptoms (McCarthy and Petrakis 2011). Integrated cognitive-behavioral therapy is more effective than individual substance counseling alone (McGovern et al. 2015).

Several such programs that encompass substance use and mental health needs have been developed, such as the Addiction and Trauma Recovery Integration Model (ATRIUM); Trauma, Addiction, Mental Health, and Recovery (TAMAR); Trauma Recovery and Empowerment Model (TREM); Trauma Affect Regulation: Guide for Education and Therapy (TARGET); and Seeking Safety. However, a trafficked person, as with any trauma victim, may still suffer from a higher burden of mental symptoms even after improvement, and maintenance treatment needs to focus on elements of anxiety sensitivity, linked to increasing likelihood to decompensate under stress (Vujanovic et al. 2018), and dissociation, which is underrecognized or misdiagnosed (Bækkelund et al. 2018). Additionally, increasing trauma severity links to psychotic symptoms, and substance use easily exacerbates these issues (Williams et al. 2018). These mental health issues may require medications to manage them even after substance abstinence has occurred.

Conversely, even with successful mental health treatment, SUDs may persist, warranting additional evidence-based treatments targeting both SUDs and mental health symptoms. Such treatments include motivational enhancement therapy, 12-step programs, and/or medication-assisted treatments. Medication-assisted treatments, particularly for opioid use disorders, are recommended and significantly increase retention in treatment (Mattick et al. 2009). Future research will need to explore the relative efficacy of SUD treatments in this especially complex population.

RETENTION IN TREATMENT AND RED FLAGS

Adherence to treatment may be a challenge for trafficked persons for many reasons. First, their other immediate needs may not have been met or stabilized at the start of their substance use treatment. Second, trafficked persons may be reluctant to engage with substance use services because of their fear of discrimination and feelings of shame about their human trafficking experiences or their substance use (Clawson and Dutch 2008). This fear and shame may be especially acute for international sex trafficking survivors, who may experience yet another level of marginalization and vulnerability.

Another important consideration is the avoidance of assumptions when working with a trafficked person. Evidence has shown that drug use often precedes someone's trafficking situation (Oram et al. 2012), although many trafficked persons note that their trafficking situation worsened their addiction as noted earlier (see section "Prevalence of Substance Use Disorders in Trafficked Persons"). In fact, Lederer and Wetzel (2014) found that among domestic sex trafficked persons, 84% reported using alcohol, drugs, or both during their period of trafficking (Lederer and Wetzel 2014). Further complicating factors include the fact that many trafficking victims are children, a population that because of ongoing development is particularly vulnerable to the effects of trauma on the brain (Levine 2017). As has been demonstrated, the structure of the brain responds to trauma and stress through changes in neuroplasticity and brain function (McEwen et al. 2015; Wilson et al. 2015); a vicious cycle of stress can increase the growing brain's vulnerability to stress from abuse (Levine 2017). Introducing substances to a growing brain further complicates the relationship between stress and brain development and may affect the appropriateness of substance use treatments for trafficked persons uniquely depending on the degree of impairment in brain function.

To be accepted into a program, patients may have to complete multiple steps in the traditional structure of substance use programs, which emphasizes substance abstinence. For trafficked persons with a concomitant SUD, those requirements can become impediments that result in both relapse and a resumption of victimization status

(Gerassi 2018). Eviction from the program may have far-reaching consequences because some individuals truly have no other place to go. Coordination between various services and some flexibility may be needed to achieve a successful treatment framework for this population (Hemmings et al. 2016).

Clinicians providing treatment for this population must have certain competencies to increase the chances of successful treatment. These competencies include general awareness of present-day immigration policies and immigration-based resources (Yakushko 2009); training in working with victims of sexual, interpersonal, and other trauma (Aron et al. 2006; Omelaniuk 2005); and the ability to work in an interdisciplinary team that may include law enforcement (Van Impe 2000). Clinicians must be mindful of comorbidities that impact treatment planning and relapse prevention. For example, individuals suffering from complex trauma related to human trafficking are also at higher risk for self-destructive and risk-taking behaviors, revictimization, and difficulties with interpersonal and intimate relationships (Courtois 2004). Finally, cultural competence and skills in working with interpreters are critical because trafficked persons have previously cited clinicians' lack of cultural appropriateness and sensitivity as the primary reason for their dissatisfaction with their mental health treatment. This may be pronounced, given the additional stigma around substance use, further highlighting the importance of a person-centered and trauma-informed approach.

BIAS, STIGMA, AND COUNTERTRANSFERENCE IN THE TREATMENT OF TRAFFICKED PERSONS WITH SUBSTANCE USE DISORDERS

Trafficked persons represent a conglomeration of difficult medical and social conditions that many clinicians dread confronting in their practices. These patients, quite unwittingly, highlight the deficiencies of health care systems—the lack of attention to social needs, the lack of evidence-based long-term effective treatments for mental illness and addiction, and the callousness of the system. Thus, trafficked persons can easily be victims of stigma and bias. As outlined in the section "Retention in Treatment and Red Flags," optimal care for this vulnerable population requires a dedicated multidisciplinary approach that is often unavailable. In this section, we will examine how care can be impacted by the feelings that clinicians harbor in the context of providing treatment. Diagnostic overshadowing and implicit bias must be kept in check to avoid misdiagnosis and mistreatment (Stoklosa et al. 2017).

Countertransference was described by Freud as a reaction that clinicians develop following interactions with their patients (Freud 1910/1957). The term most commonly used to describe negative feelings from clinicians to patients in modern medical settings includes stigma and bias, although countertransference is far more nuanced descriptively and may be more useful in educational and practical endeavors, as it conveys less prejudice.

Data on negative feelings toward mental health patients abound. In everyday medical care, patients with SUDs feel undervalued and undesired, to the point of avoiding seemingly unrelated medical areas, such as dental care (Brondani et al. 2017). Emergency physicians and internists in general feel unprepared and mostly unwilling and unexcited to take care of patients with SUDs (Mendiola et al. 2018; Wakeman et al. 2016). Moreover, for patients with combined SUDs and mental illness, negative attitudes run deep as well, starting in residency (Avery et al. 2019). Training in culturally sensitive perspectives helps but remains underutilized (Haider et al. 2015; Nelson et al. 2015).

The challenge associated with negative countertransference toward patients is that trafficked patients may present decisional dilemmas that are difficult for clinicians to navigate, thus exposing the patient to the possibility of missed treatment opportunities. For instance, the literature establishes quite clearly that trafficked persons are often victims of violence and may come to emergency departments for related injuries. Yet the literature also indicates that the reporting of intimate partner violence or domestic violence to the police—and the corresponding admission rates—is racially (Tol et al. 2019) and socioeconomically biased (Lipsky et al. 2009).

A useful way to classify countertransference is outlined in the seminal paper by Betan et al. (2005), in which eight dimensions of countertransference experienced by clinicians are described as co-occurring to various extents when dealing with patients: 1) overwhelmed/disorganized, 2) helpless/inadequate, 3) positive, 4) special/overinvolved, 5) sexualized, 6) disengaged, 7) parental/protective, and 8) criticized/mistreated.

The types of countertransference elicited by trafficked persons can be as variable as the types of individuals interviewing the patients. However, we draw attention to feeling overwhelmed (most patients will present with complex histories), feeling helpless/inadequate (social needs are often inadequately addressed and difficult to fix), and feeling overly protective (this may increase the risk of burn-out in clinicians). In addition, trauma often leads to development of borderline personality features, which can manifest in unpleasant or stressful encounters in the medical setting (Yalch and Levendosky 2019), and borderline traits and personality disorders are highly associated with SUDs as well (Kienast et al. 2014). Thus, in the clinical encounter, especially in acute settings, clinicians may feel criticized and mistreated. Addressing these feelings and adhering to treatment algorithms, as well as seeking support from colleagues, may greatly improve clinicians' coping with such challenging patients.

Pearls and Pointers

- Substance use disorders (SUDs) are very common in trafficked persons. Some victims are substance users prior to being trafficked, but the trafficking experience worsens the addictive behaviors.

- Substance use contributes to mental and physical health sequelae of human trafficking, and integrated multidisciplinary treatment is needed for positive outcomes.

- Some tenets of addiction treatment may exacerbate human trafficking struggles, especially homelessness. Housing and safety must be the first goals.

- Medication-assisted treatment for SUDs and careful management of mental illness are needed, often on a long-term basis.

- Clinicians can expect to develop strong feelings of countertransference and some bias and prejudice toward this patient population; these feelings need to be addressed both as a learning experience and a means to provide truly effective interventions.

REFERENCES

American Psychiatric Association: Diagnostic and Statistical Manual of Mental Disorders, 5th Edition. Arlington, VA, American Psychiatric Association, 2013

Aron LY, Zweig JM, Newmark LC: Comprehensive services for survivors of human trafficking: findings from clients in three communities. 2006. Available at: www.urban.org/sites/default/files/publication/43051/411507-Comprehensive-Services-for-Survivors-of-Human-Trafficking.PDF. Accessed November 5, 2019.

Avery JD, Taylor KE, Kast KA, et al: Attitudes toward individuals with mental illness and substance use disorders among resident physicians. Prim Care Companion CNS Disord 21(1):18m02382, 2019 30620451

Bækkelund H, Frewen P, Lanius R, et al: Trauma-related altered states of consciousness in post-traumatic stress disorder patients with or without comorbid dissociative disorders. Eur J Psychotraumatol 9(1):1544025, 2018 30455853

Betan E, Heim AK, Zittel Conklin C, et al: Countertransference phenomena and personality pathology in clinical practice: an empirical investigation. Am J Psychiatry 162(5):890–898, 2005 15863790

Brondani MA, Alan R, Donnelly L: Stigma of addiction and mental illness in healthcare: the case of patients' experiences in dental settings. PLoS One 12(5):e0177388, 2017 28531176

Caliber: Evaluation of comprehensive services for victims of human trafficking: key findings and lessons learned. June 2007. Available at: www.ncjrs.gov/pdffiles1/nij/grants/218777.pdf. Accessed November 5, 2019.

Clawson HJ, Dutch N: Identifying victims of human trafficking: inherent challenges and promising strategies from the field. January 20, 2008. Available at: https://aspe.hhs.gov/report/identifying-victims-human-trafficking-inherent-challenges-and-promising-strategies-field. Accessed November 5, 2019.

Clawson HJ, Dutch N, Solomon A, et al: Human trafficking into and within the United States: a review of the literature. Office of the Assistant Secretary for Planning and Evaluation, August 30, 2009. Available at: https://aspe.hhs.gov/report/human-trafficking-and-within-united-states-review-literature. Accessed November 5, 2019.

Cook MC, Barnert E, Ijadi-Maghsoodi R, et al: Exploring mental health and substance use treatment needs of commercially sexually exploited youth participating in a specialty juvenile court. Behav Med 44(3):242–249, 2018 29558256

Courtois C: Complex trauma, complex reactions: assessment and treatment. Psychotherapy: Theory, Research, Practice, Training 41(4):412–425, 2004

Farley M, Cotton A, Lynne J, et al: Prostitution and trafficking in nine countries. Journal of Trauma Practice 2(3–4):33–74, 2004

Freud S:.The future prospects of psycho-analytic therapy (1910), in Standard Edition of the Complete Psychological Works of Sigmund Freud, Vol XI. London, Hogarth Press, 1957

Gerassi LB: Barriers to accessing detox facilities, substance use treatment, and residential services among women impacted by commercial sexual exploitation and trafficking. Behav Med 44(3):199–208, 2018 28985156

Gibbons P, Stoklosa H: Identification and treatment of human trafficking victims in the emergency department: a case report. J Emerg Med 50(5):715–719, 2016 26896287

Goldberg AP, Moore JL, Houck C, et al: Domestic minor sex trafficking patients: a retrospective analysis of medical presentation. J Pediatr Adolesc Gynecol 30(1):109–115, 2017 27575407

Haider AH, Schneider EB, Sriram N, et al: Unconscious race and social class bias among acute care surgical clinicians and clinical treatment decisions. JAMA Surg 150(5):457–464, 2015 25786199

Hemmings S, Jakobowitz S, Abas M, et al: Responding to the health needs of survivors of human trafficking: a systematic review. BMC Health Serv Res 16:320, 2016 27473258

Kienast T, Stoffers J, Bermpohl F, et al: Borderline personality disorder and comorbid addiction: epidemiology and treatment. Dtsch Arztebl Int 111(16):280–286, 2014 24791755

Landers M, McGrath K, Johnson MH, et al: Baseline characteristics of dependent youth who have been commercially sexually exploited: findings from a specialized treatment program. J Child Sex Abus 26(6):692–709, 2017 28656806

Le PD, Ryan N, Rosenstock Y, et al: Health issues associated with commercial sexual exploitation and sex trafficking of children in the United States: a systematic review. Behav Med 44(3):219–233, 2018 30020867

Lederer LJ, Wetzel CA: The health consequences of sex trafficking and their implications for identifying victims in healthcare facilities. Annals of Health Law 23(1):61–87, 2014

Levine JA: Mental health issues in survivors of sex trafficking. Cogent Medicine 4(1):1278841, 2017

Lipsky S, Caetano R, Roy-Byrne P: Racial and ethnic disparities in police-reported intimate partner violence and risk of hospitalization among women. Womens Health Issues 19(2):109–118, 2009 19272561

Macy RJ, Johns N: Aftercare services for international sex trafficking survivors: informing U.S. service and program development in an emerging practice area. Trauma Violence Abuse 12(2):87–98, 2011 21196435

Mattick RP, Breen C, Kimber J, et al: Methadone maintenance therapy versus no opioid replacement therapy for opioid dependence. Cochrane Database Syst Rev (3):CD002209, 2009 19588333

McCarthy E, Petrakis I: Case report on the use of cognitive processing therapy-cognitive, enhanced to address heavy alcohol use. J Trauma Stress 24(4):474–478, 2011 21780191

McEwen BS, Gray J, Nasca C: Recognizing resilience: learning from the effects of stress on the brain. Neurobiol Stress 1:1–11, 2015 25506601

McGovern MP, Lambert-Harris C, Xie H, et al: A randomized controlled trial of treatments for co-occurring substance use disorders and post-traumatic stress disorder. Addiction 110(7):1194–1204, 2015 25846251

Mendiola CK, Galetto G, Fingerhood M: An exploration of emergency physicians' attitudes toward patients with substance use disorder. J Addict Med 12(2):132–135, 2018 29351141

Moore JL, Houck C, Hirway P, et al: Trafficking experiences and psychosocial features of domestic minor sex trafficking victims. J Interpers Violence 886260517703373, Apr 1, 2017 29294728

Nelson SC, Prasad S, Hackman HW: Training providers on issues of race and racism improve health care equity. Pediatr Blood Cancer 62(5):915–917, 2015 25683782

Omelaniuk I: Gender, poverty reduction, and migration. 2005. Available at: https://pdfs.semanticscholar.org/760f/5a843f9af4f7f515fc114f9025dff494b9a5.pdf?_ga=2.129023564.1579682066.1572995300-586094439.1572460066. Accessed November 5, 2019.

Oram S, Stöckl H, Busza J, et al: Prevalence and risk of violence and the physical, mental, and sexual health problems associated with human trafficking: systematic review. PLoS Med 9(5):e1001224, 2012 22666182

Oram S, Abas M, Bick D, et al: Human trafficking and health: a survey of male and female survivors in England. Am J Public Health 106(6):1073–1078, 2016 27077341

Raymond JG, Hughes DM: Sex trafficking of women in the United States: international and domestic trends. April 17, 2001. Available at: https://pdfs.semanticscholar.org/760f/5a843f9af4f7f515fc114f9025dff494b9a5.pdf?_ga=2.129023564.1579682066.1572995300-586094439.1572460066. Accessed November 5, 2019.

Reid JA, Piquero AR: On the relationships between commercial sexual exploitation/prostitution, substance dependency, and delinquency in youthful offenders. Child Maltreat 19(3–4):247–260, 2014 24920248

Shandro J, Chisolm-Straker M, Duber HC, et al: Human trafficking: a guide to identification and approach for the emergency physician. Ann Emerg Med 68(4):501.e1–508.e1, 2016 27130802

Stoklosa H: Anti-trafficking policy developments impacting health care providers. March 29, 2016. Available at: www.acf.hhs.gov/archive/otip/resource/stoklosa. Accessed November 5, 2019.

Stoklosa H, MacGibbon M, Stoklosa J: Human trafficking, mental illness, and addiction: avoiding diagnostic overshadowing. AMA J Ethics 19(1):23–34, 2017 28107153

Tol WA, Murray SM, Lund C, et al: Can mental health treatments help prevent or reduce intimate partner violence in low- and middle-income countries? A systematic review. BMC Womens Health 19(1):34, 2019 30764813

U.S. Department of Justice: Massachusetts man sentenced to 17 years for sex trafficking women by exploiting their opioid addictions. Justice News, December 6, 2018. Available at: www.justice.gov/opa/pr/massachusetts-man-sentenced-17-years-sex-trafficking-women-exploiting-their-opioid-addictions. Accessed November 5, 2019.

Van Impe K: People for sale: the need for a multidisciplinary approach towards human trafficking. Int Migr 38(3):113–131, 2000 12296139

Varma S, Gillespie S, McCracken C, et al: Characteristics of child commercial sexual exploitation and sex trafficking victims presenting for medical care in the United States. Child Abuse Negl 44:98–105, 2015 25896617

Vujanovic AA, Farris SG, Bartlett BA, et al: Anxiety sensitivity in the association between posttraumatic stress and substance use disorders: a systematic review. Clin Psychol Rev 62:37–55, 2018 29778929

Wakeman SE, Pham-Kanter G, Donelan K: Attitudes, practices, and preparedness to care for patients with substance use disorder: results from a survey of general internists. Subst Abus 37(4):635–641, 2016 27164025

Williams J, Bucci S, Berry K, et al: Psychological mediators of the association between childhood adversities and psychosis: a systematic review. Clin Psychol Rev 65:175–196, 2018 30243100

Wilson MA, Grillo CA, Fadel JR, et al: Stress as a one-armed bandit: differential effects of stress paradigms on the morphology, neurochemistry and behavior in the rodent amygdala. Neurobiol Stress 1:195–208, 2015 26844236

Yakushko O: Human trafficking: a review for mental health professionals. Int J Adv Couns 31(3):158–167, 2009

Yalch MM, Levendosky AA: Influence of betrayal trauma on borderline personality disorder traits. J Trauma Dissociation 20(4):392–401, 2019 30681038

CHAPTER 10

General and Specific Psychotherapy Considerations for Managing Trafficked Adults

Temilola Salami, Ph.D.

Grace Boland, B.A.

Christina Engelken, M.A.

> Courage doesn't always roar. Sometimes courage is the little voice at the end of the day that says I'll try again tomorrow.
>
> —*Mary Anne Radmacher, Survivor*

> This is how I am rebuilding my life, one page at a time, one day at a time.
>
> —*Amanda Berry, Survivor*

Force, fraud, and coercion are methods used by traffickers to enslave, entrap, and exploit trafficked persons for their own gain (United Nations Office of Drugs and Crime 2014). For those who escape servitude, the trauma of their trafficked experience may continue to cause pain and suffering (Banović and Bjelajac 2012; Le 2017; Mohr 2017; Pascual-Leone et al. 2017; Ravi et al. 2017; Sukach et al. 2018). Trafficked persons will likely need the aid of psychological services to enable them to adequately process trauma experiences and to decrease the adverse psychological consequences resulting from their trafficked experience. Although trafficked persons are a diverse group of people from different socioeconomic and demographic backgrounds (Bennett-Murphy 2012; Pascual-Leone et al. 2017), their unique experience of being trafficked necessitates specific treatment considerations. Mental health professionals must be aware of possible symptom manifestations within this group and how best to aid this population.

In this chapter, we aim to outline intra-individual and extra-individual factors that are pertinent to consider when working with trafficked persons. We propose that considering these factors in clinical care will enable mental health professionals to be more aware and sensitive to the needs of victims and help strengthen the therapeutic alliance. Tables 10–1 and 10–2 summarize some of the key considerations discussed in detail in the remainder of the chapter. It is important to note that although forced labor is estimated to be more widespread than sex trafficking, much of the existing literature is focused on victims of human sex trafficking (Yakushko 2009). For this reason, much of our discussion stems from research conducted with sex-trafficked adults.

INTRA-INDIVIDUAL FACTORS

Intra-individual factors may serve to promote or hinder treatment progress and represent patient factors that mental health professionals would need to assess for treatment to be successful (Cary et al. 2016; Pascual-Leone et al. 2017). For trafficked persons, these factors may have been present prior to being trafficked or developed as a result of being trafficked. Trafficked persons in mental health settings will likely be viewed as patients; hereafter, trafficked persons and patient will be used interchangeably. We now discuss a number of factors that therapists should consider when working with trafficked persons (see Table 10–1 for a summary of these factors).

Trust

As a result of the forceful, fraudulent, and coercive tactics used by traffickers to dominate and compel trafficked persons into compliance, trafficked persons may not be readily trusting of others, including those in the helping professions (Hemmings et al. 2016; Hom and Woods 2013; Hopper 2017; Orme and Ross-Sheriff 2015; Pascual-Leone et al. 2017; Preble 2015). Distrust in this population is likely protective as trafficked persons may fear retaliation for speaking out against their traffickers (Hemmings et al. 2016; Hopper 2017; Preble 2015). For trafficked persons to safely speak out against their abusers, they must be believed, fully protected, and provided with adequate services. If they speak out and these conditions are not met, trafficked persons may be at risk of revictimization by resentful traffickers. As a result of these fears and distrust, trafficked persons may initially present as hostile, resistant, or indifferent toward their medical care

TABLE 10-1. Summary of treatment considerations for intra-individual factors

INTRA-INDIVIDUAL FACTORS	POSTTRAFFICKING CONSIDERATIONS	HOW HEALTH PROFESSIONALS CAN INTERVENE
Trust	Distrust of others	Believe, protect, and provide patients appropriate services.
	Limited disclosure	Build a safe and supportive environment.
		Educate patients about privacy and confidentiality.
		Educate patients about the course of therapy and dispel misconceptions about therapy.
Attachment	Attachment and interpersonal difficulties	Acknowledge and normalize ambivalence toward traffickers.
		Emphasize autonomy.
		Help patients form healthy attachments.
		Set clear boundaries and roles.
Psychological status	Internalizing symptoms (e.g., low self-esteem, hopelessness, shame)	Assess for psychological symptoms associated with trauma.
	Externalizing symptoms (e.g., rage, aggression)	Conduct crisis stabilization prior to beginning treatment.
	Negative view of one's self, world, and future	Help patients develop adaptive coping skills.
		Assess for both primary and secondary emotions and help trafficked persons process these emotions.
		Increase hope.
		Promote self-esteem through challenging negative beliefs, increasing assertiveness, and building strengths (Hopper 2017).

(Hemmings et al. 2016; Hopper 2017; Pascual-Leone et al. 2017). In addition to providing a safe and supportive environment for trafficked persons, mental health professionals need to educate patients about the rules related to privacy and confidentiality (Ravi et al. 2017). Furthermore, as a means of building trust, rapport, and transparency, mental health professionals should take the time to educate patients about their role as therapists and inform patients about what to expect from therapy (Cecchet and Thoburn 2014; Chung 2009). Patients' expectations of therapy should be discussed, and any misconceptions that patients may have about the course of therapy should be clarified.

Because of the importance of trust in the therapeutic setting, we have included a brief review of a case study conducted by Napoli et al. (2001). Napoli and colleagues expounded on the case of "Bonnie," a former prostitute. On the basis of the information provided by Napoli and colleagues, Bonnie is not a victim of trafficking because her situation did not include force, fraud, or coercion; however, her concerns are likely similar to those of trafficked persons. Bonnie was a survivor of incestuous sexual abuse and began prostituting herself at the age of 16. Nine years later, at the age of 25, she sought treatment and discussed her internal struggle about seeking treatment. She stated the following:

> I was afraid to go into therapy because I expected to get emotionally beat up. I thought I'd have to hear all about everything that was wrong with me and how bad and messed up I was…I was very surprised when my therapist began by validating and praising me for being willing to address the things that lead me to prostitution. I craved affirmation. I think that's why I kept going back…. As a child I waited for someone to come and save me. Eventually I gave up and after that the thought never occurred to me again. Now, amazingly, I was getting what I always wanted and had long ago given up looking for. For the first time I got to hear someone to say, "That was wrong! You were a precious little girl who deserved much, much better!" And I began to learn how to reparent myself. I learned how to love and not abuse myself. (Napoli et al. 2001)

The intra-individual factor of distrust of the therapist was initially a barrier to Bonnie's treatment. Preconceived notions about therapy, past difficult experiences with authority figures, and prior sexual abuse, particularly by family members, can all influence feelings of mistrust toward caregivers. As illustrated by Bonnie's case, these are important factors to be aware of and address in the therapeutic setting to enhance rapport and treatment engagement. Napoli and colleagues (2001) recommend consistent acceptance and support, as well as helping the client articulate the reasons for his or her resistance to treatment to help normalize and overcome this barrier.

Attachment

Through the use of manipulative and coercive tactics (e.g., convincing trafficked persons that they are in a romantic relationship with their trafficker) or as a result of familial ties, some trafficked persons may have formed emotional attachments to their traffickers (Pascual-Leone et al. 2017). This is a normative experience and one that may have been purposefully cultivated by traffickers to keep trafficked persons fully dependent on them for basic needs (e.g., food, shelter, emotional support). Thus, in the therapeutic setting, mental health professionals may face the challenge of trafficked persons not identifying themselves as victims, fearing to speak out against their traffickers, or having ambivalent emotional reactions toward their traffickers (Orme and Ross-Sheriff 2015; Pascual-Leone et al. 2017). This ambivalence may mean seeing traffickers as parental or romantic figures whom one has loving feelings toward and seeing traffickers as enslavers and exploiters (Orme and Ross-Sheriff 2015). Normalizing, acknowledging, and working through this ambivalence may result in decreased emotional distress among trafficked persons.

Past abuse in childhood, and negative interpersonal relationships, put individuals at risk for exploitation (O'Brien 2018). Thus, trafficked persons must learn to develop nonexploitative, healthy, and positive relationships. As a means of decreasing vulnerability to revictimization, mental health professionals can educate trafficked persons about the process of trafficking and the various tactics traffickers use to develop emotional attachments (e.g., fear, threats, isolation, manipulation, affection, dependency). The patient's emotional needs may affect the therapeutic relationship because mental health professionals may be perceived as new authority figures and surrogates for trafficked persons' past relationships with traffickers (Kleinschmidt 2009). Therapists will need to strive to gain patients' trust, a crucial element of therapeutic work with trafficked persons. Therapists will also need to set clear boundaries and roles, emphasize the patient's autonomy and independence, and help patients identify and form healthy attachments.

Psychological Status

Psychological factors are important to consider when working with trafficked persons because psychiatric patients are particularly vulnerable to trafficking and may experience exacerbation of symptoms as a result of being trafficked (Cary et al. 2016). Psychological symptoms such as depression, anxiety, psychosis, and trauma symptoms acquired both pretrafficking and posttrafficking can have a significant impact on treatment outcomes (Hopper 2017). Thus, mental health professionals should work to better understand the onset, course, and maintenance of psychological symptoms for this population. Self-esteem is one vulnerability factor to consider as lower levels of self-esteem increase vulnerability to being trafficked (Hopper 2017; Ravi et al. 2017; Sukach et al. 2018). However, it is important to note that low self-esteem is neither necessary nor sufficient to being trafficked. Furthermore, individuals who are victims of trafficking may experience a decline in self-esteem (Sukach et al. 2018). Promoting self-esteem through challenging negative beliefs, engaging in assertiveness training, and building on patients' strengths may be needed in the therapy setting (Hopper 2017).

Other emotional reactions that can result from being trafficked include feelings of hopelessness (Sukach et al. 2018), shame (Contreras et al. 2017; Hom and Woods 2013), and more externalized emotions such as rage and aggression (Bennett-Murphy 2012). Furthermore, a change in how one views himself or herself, the world, and the future can result from being trafficked (Pascual-Leone et al. 2017). This shift in perspective may influence emotional reactions and impact psychological health (Logan et al. 2009; Pascual-Leone et al. 2017; Salami et al. 2018). Posttrafficking, trafficked persons may come to view the world as unjust, view people as inherently evil, or believe themselves to be unsafe (Pascual-Leone et al. 2017).

Depending on the intensity, the aforementioned emotional reactions and changes in basic life assumptions may mark the presence of PTSD, depression, or other deleterious psychological consequences of trauma such as self-harm behaviors (Banović and Bjelajac 2012; Logan et al. 2009; Pascual-Leone et al. 2017; Salami et al. 2018). Maladaptive coping strategies as a means of numbing or avoiding psychological pain, such as parasuicidal behaviors or substance use, may be particularly common among human trafficking victims (Banović and Bjelajac 2012; Ravi et al. 2017; Sukach et al. 2018). Given the evidence for *multifinality* (i.e., similar exposure to trauma may lead to different psychological outcomes; Banović and Bjelajac 2012; Hopper 2017; Okech et al. 2018), mental health professionals should comprehensively assess for different psychological symptoms that may result from trauma. Mental health professionals should be aware that treatment seeking may differ among trafficked persons, with a variety of factors, including distrust (Ravi et al. 2017), fear of their trafficker (Hemmings et al. 2016; Hom and Woods 2013; Hopper 2017; Orme and Ross-Sheriff 2015; Pascual-Leone et al. 2017; Preble 2015), and fear of stigma or hopelessness, impacting patients' motivation for change (Sukach et al. 2018). Assessing readiness for change, perhaps by using a motivational interviewing framework (Wirsing 2012), might be an important first step for conceptualizing the case, building rapport, and effecting symptom relief.

It is imperative that mental health professionals assess for both primary and secondary emotions that trafficked persons experience as a result of their trafficked experience and work to process these emotions, providing relief through replacement of maladaptive coping skills (e.g., self-harm) with more adaptive coping skills (Abas et al. 2013; Okech et al. 2018; Ravi et al. 2017). Mental health professionals should communicate messages of hope to trafficked persons, letting them know that there is life after trafficking and that their psychological symptoms can be reduced with available treatments (Sukach et al. 2018). Furthermore, psychiatric crisis intervention may be necessary for some patients. Mental health professionals should assess the need for crisis stabilization prior to beginning therapy (Gibbs et al. 2015; Orme and Ross-Sheriff 2015; Pascual-Leone et al. 2017).

EXTRA-INDIVIDUAL FACTORS

Extra-individual factors are extrinsic to the individual yet have influence on the onset and course of patients' symptoms, as well as their access to care (Ijadi-Maghsoodi et al. 2018; Meshkovska et al. 2015; Sukach et al. 2018). Trafficked persons have a multitude of extrinsic obstacles that impede their ability to seek and receive adequate mental health services. We will discuss some of these factors in this section (see Table 10–2 for a summary of these factors).

Stigma

For victims of sex trafficking, perhaps the biggest obstacle to seeking and receiving adequate mental health services is the stigma associated with sex work (Dahal et al. 2015; Weitzer 2018). The criminalization of prostitution by the criminal justice system has resulted in trafficked persons being marginalized by society (Vanwesenbeeck 2017). Indeed, trafficked persons are often arrested for prostitution while perpetrators remain unidentified (Primrose 2011). Because

TABLE 10-2. Summary of treatment considerations for extra-individual factors

EXTRA-INDIVIDUAL FACTORS	POSTTRAFFICKING CONSIDERATIONS	HOW HEALTH PROFESSIONALS CAN INTERVENE
Stigma	Stigmatized/ marginalized	Dispel human trafficking myths and misconceptions, paying attention to your own biases.
Supportive networks	Victim isolation	Connect trafficked persons with families.
		Help patients identify and develop supportive networks.
		With the aid of social workers, help clients reintegrate into safe communities.
Socioeconomic barriers	Social, economic, and legal instability	Be aware of programs and laws relevant to patients.
		Connect trafficked persons to appropriate programs.
		Consult with social workers.
		Help trafficked persons become self-reliant and self-sufficient.
Identification	Lack of self-identification	Use available screening tools to help identify trafficked persons.
	Lack of training among mental health professionals	When possible, assess patients alone.
	Language and cultural barriers	Use interpreters when possible.
		Provide information about where patients can seek help or further assistance.

TABLE 10-2. Summary of treatment considerations for extra-individual factors *(continued)*

EXTRA-INDIVIDUAL FACTORS	POSTTRAFFICKING CONSIDERATIONS	HOW HEALTH PROFESSIONALS CAN INTERVENE
Therapist competence	Potential biases and assumptions about clients	Strive toward greater clinical and multicultural competence.
	Lack of training in mental health care of trafficked persons	Be aware of boundaries of competence.
		Consult and refer when appropriate.

fear prevents individuals from reporting their abusers, trafficked persons rather than perpetrators are convicted and prosecuted (Adams 2011). Prosecution may lead to downward social mobility as it becomes more difficult for trafficked persons with criminal convictions to access stable employment, education, and housing (Barnard 2014; Bocinski 2017; Solomon 2012). This in turn contributes to negative mental health outcomes that can further perpetuate a downward socioeconomic drift (Bocinski 2017; Busch-Armendariz et al. 2016; Dank et al. 2017; Meshkovska et al. 2015). For these reasons, it is pertinent that clinicians who are invested in working with trafficked persons provide law enforcement agencies with psychoeducation about who the victims are and work with law enforcement and other stakeholders (e.g., social workers) to promote victim-centered care (Yakushko 2009). Both trafficked persons and health care professionals may hold negative beliefs about human trafficking victims (Sukach et al. 2018); mental health professionals should be aware of and work to combat their own biases and underlying judgments prior to working with trafficked persons.

Supportive Networks

Trafficked persons may have been forced or coerced to engage in illegal or culturally taboo activity during their capture (Bennett-Murphy 2012; Mohr 2017), and thus they may be perceived negatively by members of their community (Zimmerman and Pocock 2013). Indeed, many trafficked persons return home to find themselves rejected by their families (Brunovskis and Surtees 2007). Others keep their experience of being trafficked a secret out of fear of being shamed, leading to tension in victims' interpersonal relationships (Brunovskis and Surtees 2013). While being trafficked, most trafficked persons' social circles are limited to traffickers, pimps, and customers (Sukach et al. 2018). As most women trafficked through the sex industry are repeatedly abused by males, many may continue to be distrusting of men and have difficulty maintaining interpersonal relationships with men posttrafficking. A generalized distrust of all males may create obstacles for trafficked persons and would need to be addressed in treatment (Dalla 2006; Domoney et al. 2015; Sukach et al. 2018).

Economic disadvantage is a push factor for trafficking (Banović and Bjelajac 2012), with some trafficked persons being forced by their families or those in their social group into labor or sex work for financial gain (Zimmerman and Pocock 2013). To create dependence and as a tactic to control trafficked persons, traffickers isolate victims from supportive friends and families and other trafficked persons. The social networks of trafficked persons are limited while they are trafficked, and posttrafficking, persons are often socially isolated (De Angelis 2014; Pascual-Leone et al. 2017). Social support increases psychological health, and positive social networks may shield trafficked persons from future victimization (Okech et al. 2018). A goal of therapy should thus be to help patients reintegrate into safe and supportive communities (Okech et al. 2018). Therapists may need to reconnect trafficked persons to supportive loved ones and help trafficked persons form healthy relationships (Judge 2018; O'Brien 2018).

Supportive contributions from family members during the recovery and treatment process can be beneficial to trafficked persons (Abas et al. 2013). However, supportive family members may have experienced vicarious trauma and may also benefit from psychological assistance. Providing such assistance to families while working to dispel potential myths and misconceptions that families might have about human trafficking can help strengthen familial bonds and enhance the recovery process for trafficked persons (Cohen et al. 2017).

Socioeconomic Barriers

According to Surtees (2010), *reintegration* is "the process of recovery involving economic and social inclusion following a trafficking experience." This process includes a stable and sustainable standard of living as well as opportunities for economic growth (Surtees 2012).

Unfortunately, reintegration may be difficult, specifically because trafficked persons often live a life of social, economic, and legal in-stability, creating a significant risk for revictimization (Adams 2011; Domoney et al. 2015). Posttrafficking, and prior to any therapeutic work, trafficked persons' basic needs (e.g., medical care, safety, hous-ing, transportation, childcare, insurance) must be assessed. In collab-oration with social workers, therapists would need to help patients move toward self-reliance and self-sufficiency by providing avenues for basic needs to be met (see Gordon et al. 2018).

Additionally, immigration is a significant obstacle many victims of human trafficking must navigate. trafficked persons who have been trafficked over international borders may face the threat of deporta-tion (Adams 2011). One important resource for trafficked persons is the T visa program, which provides a potential path to citizenship for victims (Barbagiannis 2017). To qualify for the T visa program, an individual must meet four criteria: 1) they must have been traf-ficked in the United States, 2) they must have been a victim of severe trafficking, 3) they must cooperate with law enforcement during the investigation and prosecution of perpetrators, and 4) they must pro-vide evidence that they will experience "undue hardship" if deported (Barbagiannis 2017). Because the T visa program is unknown to many trafficked persons, it is important that clinicians become fa-miliar with this program and provide victims with the necessary in-formation (Todd 2017).

Identification

Trafficked persons may be burdened by medical concerns (e.g., infec-tious diseases, pregnancy, and injuries due to abuse or unsafe work-ing environments) and psychiatric concerns (e.g., overdose, psychosis, withdrawal symptoms) that necessitate medical intervention (Oram et al. 2012; Orme and Ross-Sheriff 2015; Ottisova et al. 2016, 2018; Pascual-Leone et al. 2017). Trafficked persons are often subject to a cyclical pattern of violence, in which they are abused and then cared for in order to ensure their cooperation (Banović and Bjelajac 2012). This cycle is only broken once a trafficked person is identified and provided with adequate assistance and protection. In fact, it has been estimated that 50%–88% of trafficked persons will come into contact with a mental health professional at least once while being trafficked (Baldwin et al. 2011; Lederer and Wetzel 2014). However, many trafficked persons go unidentified and are difficult to identify for a variety of reasons. Language and cultural barriers may influence trafficked persons' understanding of their rights in foreign countries and prevent them from seeking help. Threats to trafficked persons' well-being and families are tactics used by traffickers to keep trafficked persons trapped in silence; thus, they may not seek help for fear that traffickers will retaliate (Hom and Woods 2013). Complicating matters, trafficked persons who have been coerced into believing they are in romantic and mutually beneficial relationships with traffickers may not identify themselves as victims, leading to a decrease in self-referrals as well as a lack of commitment to treatment (Cecchet and Thoburn 2014; Clawson et al. 2009; Gibbs et al. 2015).

Mental health professionals are not always well trained in victim identification, and the lack of validated and distributed screening tools in mental health settings hinders victim identification (Hemmings et al. 2016). Although not validated, screening tools have been created for health care settings. These include the Medical Assessment Tool (Polaris Project 2010) and the Screening Tool for Victims of Human Trafficking (U.S. Department of Health and Human Services 2019). Both of these tools are short screening tools that may enable mental health professionals to identify trafficked persons in health care settings. At the very least, and whenever possible, mental health professionals should screen potential trafficked persons alone and provide them with information about were to seek help. Care should be taken not to make trafficked persons' circumstances worse. Victim identification is the first step toward adequate care, with fragmented care leading to a greater possibility of revictimization (Judge 2018). Because trafficked persons are a heterogeneous group, their needs may be quite diverse and often require complex coordinated actions by programs. Trafficked persons may also require emotional stabilization and access to both physical and mental health care in addition to social work involvement and legal counsel (Banović and Bjelajac 2012; Oram et al. 2012; Ottisova et al. 2016, 2018). Mental health professionals are well suited to connect the various stakeholders in support of proper care of trafficked persons (Salami et al. 2018).

Therapist Competence

A therapist's training, self-efficacy, and competency are integral for adequate treatment of human trafficking victims (Thompson and Haley 2018; Yakushko 2009). Because trafficked persons come from different backgrounds, to better aid this diverse group the mental

health professional will need to engage in culturally competent practice (Harding-Jones 2018; Le 2017). Mental health professionals
should work to understand their own biases and assumptions, respect
cultural norms and values, gain knowledge about policies and laws
that effect trafficked persons, and develop skills to work with this
heterogeneous population (Harding-Jones 2018; Hemmings et al.
2016; Kleinschmidt 2009; Sukach et al. 2018; Yakushko 2009). Mental health professionals should become familiar with guidelines for
working with diverse populations (see Kleinschmidt 2009) and guidelines for working with trafficked persons (see Pascual-Leone et al.
2017). Since competency is a process and not an end point, mental
health professionals should continue to build on their competence
(Thompson and Haley 2018).

There remains a dearth of research on the efficacy of trauma treatments for trafficked persons. Patients may, however, benefit from
therapy approaches that have been found to be effective for other
trauma populations. Cognitive therapies (i.e., cognitive processing
therapy) and exposure therapies (i.e., prolonged exposure therapy)
are empirically supported treatments that may be well suited for
this population (see Salami et al. 2018). It is important to note, however, that cultural adaptations of these therapies may be needed for
diverse groups. In addition, narrative exposure therapy has been found
to be a helpful treatment of PTSD among trafficked persons (Robjant
et al. 2017), and it has been conditionally recommended for the treatment of PTSD among immigrant and refugee populations (American
Psychological Association 2017). Adhering to the standards of evidence-based practice, in addition to cultural competence and clinical
expertise, treatment choice should be based on the best available evidence and patient preference (Gibbs et al. 2015).

Part of engaging in competent care is knowing one's limits of competence and when to consult or refer patients to other providers (Harding-
Jones 2018). To better understand the needs of trafficked persons, a
thorough clinical assessment should be conducted (Abas et al. 2013;
Hemmings et al. 2016), with a treatment plan developed based on
the needs of the patient. Poor communication between mental health
professionals and patients limits the effectiveness of treatment
(Harding-Jones 2018). Thus, building rapport and a strong therapeutic alliance is essential for the promotion of treatment effectiveness
(Harding-Jones 2018). Considerations such as interviewing victims
in private and using trained interpreters for trafficked persons who
may speak a different language will improve the therapeutic relation-

ship and communication between therapist and patient (Hemmings et al. 2016).

Given that trafficked persons are placed in subordinate roles while being trafficked, it is important to work to build trafficked persons' sense of self-efficacy and empowerment by allowing them to be active participants in their care (Harding-Jones 2018; Sukach et al. 2018). According to Judge (2018, p. 287), mental health programs for trafficked persons must be "flexible, accessible, trauma informed, survivor driven, responsive to stages of change, multidisciplinary, and enduring." Group therapy may be especially useful in reducing shame and stigma as it gives individuals the opportunity to share their experiences with others who have endured similar trauma (Hickle and Roe-Sepowitz 2014). However, providers should be cautious about using group therapy with trafficked persons. Trafficked persons may have been forced to compete with or abuse others during their trafficking experience and may fear judgment or hostility in a group therapy environment (Salami et al. 2018; Yakushko 2009). Thus, it is important for the clinician and patient to work collaboratively on a treatment plan that will best meet the individual's needs. Continuity of care is vital for patients' psychological health and reintegration (De Angelis 2014; Okech et al. 2018). Aftercare services must be trauma sensitive, and clinicians and social workers must be knowledgeable and sensitive to the needs of their patients (Hemmings et al. 2016; Johnson 2012).

CONCLUSION

The trauma associated with human trafficking often results in a multitude of adverse psychological consequences. Because exploited individuals often do not identify themselves as victims, trafficked persons may lack the motivation to leave their situation, and identification of victims in the health care setting may be difficult. Once identified, trafficked persons may need to be connected with mental health professionals as a means of fostering motivation, decreasing trauma symptoms, and promoting successful reintegration.

As human trafficking is a unique trauma experience, special treatment considerations should be put into practice for this population. When working with trafficked persons, mental health professionals should consider both intra- and extra-individual factors that may impact the therapeutic process. Regarding intra-individual factors, mental health professionals should assess the trafficked persons' attachment to their abuser, current psychological symptoms, and level of trust. Additionally, mental health professionals should be aware of the many extra-individual factors that might impact treatment, such as stigma, the trafficked person's social support system, and socioeconomic barriers.

Perhaps most importantly, clinicians working with trafficked persons should be aware of their own limitations. Mental health workers must continuously strive to increase their competence in their work with trafficked populations. Additionally, working with trafficked persons may induce secondary traumatic stress. For this reason, consultation and supervision for less experienced clinicians is of the utmost importance. Furthermore, interdisciplinary consultation is highly recommended. For successful recovery, treatment should be flexible, culturally sensitive, continuous, and trauma informed. Without stable and adequate mental health care, as well as continuity of care, survivors are at risk for revictimization.

Pearls and Pointers

- Mental health professionals must be aware of the different intra- and extra-individual factors that are unique to trafficked persons and that can influence identification, treatment, and recovery.

- Building trust, self-efficacy, self-esteem, empowerment, and support is important to providing proper treatment for trafficked persons.

- Mental health professionals and therapists should assist trafficked persons in gaining independence and encourage these individuals to be active in their own care.

- Overcoming the stigma and biases surrounding human trafficking held by society, law enforcement officers, mental health professionals, the individual therapist, and the trafficked persons themselves is integral to identification and optimal treatment.

- Mental health professionals must strive to be competent, with an awareness of cultural factors, evidence-based treatments, and specific treatment guidelines pertinent to trafficked persons.

REFERENCES

Abas M, Ostrovschi NV, Prince M, et al: Risk factors for mental disorders in women survivors of human trafficking: a historical cohort study. BMC Psychiatry 13(1):204, 2013 23914952

Adams C: Re-trafficked victims: how a human rights approach can stop the cycle of re-victimization of sex trafficking victims. George Washington International Law Review 43(1):201–234, 2011

American Psychological Association: Clinical practice guideline for the treatment of PTSD. February 24, 2017. Available at: www.apa.org/ptsd-guideline/ptsd.pdf. Accessed November 6, 2019.

Baldwin SB, Eisenman DP, Sayles JN, et al: Identification of human trafficking victims in health care settings. Health Hum Rights 13(1):E36–E49, 2011 22772961

Banović B, Bjelajac Ž: Traumatic experiences, psychophysical consequences and needs of human trafficking victims. Vojnosanit Pregl 69(1):94–97, 2012 22397304

Barbagiannis E: Protecting victims of human trafficking: creating better residency visas. Cordozo Journal for International and Comparative Law 25(3):561–593, 2017

Barnard AM: "The second chance they deserve": vacating convictions of sex trafficking victims. Columbia Law Rev 114:1463–1501, 2014

Bennett-Murphy LM: Haunted: treatment of a child survivor of human trafficking. Journal of Infant, Child, and Adolescent Psychotherapy 11(2):133–148, 2012

Bocinski SG: The economic drivers and consequences of sex trafficking in the United States. Institute for Women's Policy Research, September 27, 2017. Available at: https://iwpr.org/publications/economic-drivers-consequences-sex-trafficking-united states/. Accessed November 6, 2019.

Brunovskis A, Surtees R: Leaving the past behind? The victims of trafficking decline assistance. Fafo, 2007. Available at: www.fafo.no/pub/rapp/20040/20040.pdf. Accessed November 6, 2019.

Brunovskis A, Surtees R: Coming home: challenges in family reintegration for trafficked women. Qualitative Social Work 12(4):454–472, 2013

Busch-Armendariz N, Nale NL, Kammer-Kerwick M, et al: Human Trafficking by the Numbers: The Initial Benchmark of Prevalence and Economic Impact for Texas. Austin, TX, Institute on Domestic Violence and Sexual Assault, The University of Texas at Austin, 2016

Cary M, Oram S, Howard LM, et al: Human trafficking and severe mental illness: an economic analysis of survivors' use of psychiatric services. BMC Health Serv Res 16(1):284, 2016 27430338

Cecchet SJ, Thoburn J: The psychological experience of child and adolescent sex trafficking in the United States: trauma and resilience in survivors. Psychological Trauma 6(5):482, 2014

Chung RCY: Cultural perspectives on child trafficking, human rights and social justice: a model for psychologists. Counselling Psychological Quarterly 22(1):85–96, 2009

Clawson HJ, Dutch NM, Solomon A, et al: Study of HHS programs serving human trafficking victims: final report, December 2009. U.S. Department of Health and Human Services, Office of the Assistant Secretary for Planning and Evaluation, 2009. Available at: http://aspc.hhs.gov/hsp/07/humantrafficking/final/index.pdf. Accessed November 6, 2019.

Cohen JA, Mannarino AP, Kinnish K: Trauma-focused cognitive behavioral therapy for commercially sexually exploited youth. J Child Adolesc Trauma 10(2):175–185, 2017 28690714

Contreras PM, Kallivayalil D, Herman JL: Psychotherapy in the aftermath of human trafficking: working through the consequences of psychological coercion. Women and Therapy 40:31–54, 2017

Dahal P, Joshi SK, Swahnberg K: "We are looked down upon and rejected socially": a qualitative study on the experiences of trafficking survivors in Nepal. Glob Health Action 8(1):29267, 2015 26584683

Dalla RL: "You can't hustle all your life": An exploratory investigation of the exit process among street-level prostituted women. Psychology of Women Quarterly 30(3):276–290, 2006

Dank M, Yahner J, Yu L: Consequences of Policing Prostitution. Washington, DC, Urban Institute, 2017

De Angelis M: "I thought I am modern slavery": giving a voice to trafficked women. British Journal of Community Justice 12(3):49–66, 2014

Domoney J, Howard LM, Abas M, et al: Mental health service responses to human trafficking: a qualitative study of professionals' experiences of providing care. BMC Psychiatry 15(1):289, 2015 26576640

Gibbs DA, Walters JLH, Lutnick A, et al: Services to domestic minor victims of sex trafficking: opportunities for engagement and support. Children and Youth Services Review 54:1–7, 2015

Gordon M, Salami T, Coverdale J, et al: Psychiatry's role in the management of human trafficking victims: an integrated care approach. J Psychiatr Pract 24(2):79–86, 2018 29509177

Harding-Jones C: Counselling sex-trafficked clients using trauma-focused cognitive behavioral therapy. Healthcare Counselling and Psychotherapy Journal 18(2):16–19, 2018

Hemmings S, Jakobowitz S, Abas M, et al: Responding to the health needs of survivors of human trafficking: a systematic review. BMC Health Serv Res 16:320, 2016 27473258

Hickle KE, Roe-Sepowitz DE: Putting the pieces back together: a group intervention for sexually exploited adolescent girls. Social Work With Groups 37(2):99–113, 2014

Hom KA, Woods SJ: Trauma and its aftermath for commercially sexually exploited women as told by front-line service providers. Issues Ment Health Nurs 34(2):75–81, 2013 23369118

Hopper EK: Trauma-informed psychological assessment of human trafficking survivors. Women and Therapy 40(1–2):12–30, 2017

Ijadi-Maghsoodi R, Bath E, Cook M, et al: Commercially sexually exploited youths' health care experiences, barriers, and recommendations: a qualitative analysis. Child Abuse Negl 76:334–341, 2018 29195171

Johnson BC: Aftercare for survivors of human trafficking. Social Work and Christianity 39(4):370–389, 2012

Judge AM: Uncharted waters: developing mental health services for survivors of domestic human sex trafficking. Harv Rev Psychiatry 26(5):287–297, 2018 30188340

Kleinschmidt L: Keeping mother alive: psychotherapy with a teenage mother following human trafficking. Journal of Child Psychotherapy 35(3):262–275, 2009

Le PD: "Reconstructing a sense of self:" trauma and coping among returned women survivors of human trafficking in Vietnam. Qual Health Res 27(4):509–519, 2017 27206456

Lederer LJ, Wetzel CA: The health consequences of sex trafficking and their implications for identifying victims in healthcare facilities. Annals of Health Law 23(1):61–87, 2014

Logan TK, Walker R, Hunt G: Understanding human trafficking in the United States. Trauma Violence Abuse 10(1):3–30, 2009 19056686

Meshkovska B, Siegel M, Stutterheim SE, et al: Female sex trafficking: conceptual issues, current debates, and future directions. J Sex Res 52(4):380–395, 2015 25897567

Mohr G: The impact of human trafficking. Corrections Today, 2017. Available at: www.aca.org/ACA_Prod_IMIS/DOCS/Corrections%20Today/2017%20Articles/November%202017/CT-Nov-Dec%202017_Trafficking.pdf. Accessed November 5, 2019.

Napoli M, Gerdes K, DeSouza-Rowland S: Treatment of prostitution using integrative therapy techniques: a case study. Journal of Contemporary Psychotherapy 31(2):71–87, 2001

O'Brien JE: "Sometimes, somebody just needs somebody—anybody—to care:" the power of interpersonal relationships in the lives of domestic minor sex trafficking survivors. Child Abuse Negl 81:1–11, 2018 29689316

Okech D, Hansen N, Howard W, et al: Social support, dysfunctional coping, and community reintegration as predictors of PTSD among human trafficking survivors. Behav Med 44(3):209–218, 2018 30020868

Oram S, Ostrovschi NV, Gorceag VI, et al: Physical health symptoms reported by trafficked women receiving post-trafficking support in Moldova: prevalence, severity and associated factors. BMC Womens Health 12(1):20, 2012 22834807

Orme J, Ross-Sheriff F: Sex trafficking: policies, programs, and services. Soc Work 60(4):287–294, 2015 26489349

Ottisova L, Hemmings S, Howard LM, et al: Prevalence and risk of violence and the mental, physical and sexual health problems associated with human trafficking: an updated systematic review. Epidemiol Psychiatr Sci 25(4):317–341, 2016 27066701

Ottisova L, Smith P, Oram S: Psychological consequences of human trafficking: Complex posttraumatic stress disorder in trafficked children. Behav Med 44(3):234–241, 2018 30020865

Pascual-Leone A, Kim J, Morrison OP: Working with victims of human trafficking. Journal of Contemporary Psychotherapy 47(1):51–59, 2017

Polaris: Medical assessment tool. 2010. Available at: https://traffickingresourcecenter.org/sites/default/files/Assessment%20Tool%20%20Medical%20Professionals.pdf. Accessed November 5, 2019.

Preble KM: Creating trust among the distrustful: a phenomenological examination of supportive services for former sex workers. Journal of Aggression, Maltreatment, and Trauma 24(4):433–453, 2015

Primrose S: Killing the messenger: the intersection between sex trafficking, planned parenthood and the marginalization of youth victims. University of Florida Journal of Law and Public Policy 22:299, 2011

Ravi A, Pfeiffer MR, Rosner Z, et al: Identifying health experiences of domestically sex-trafficked women in the USA: a qualitative study in Rikers Island jail. J Urban Health 94(3):408–416, 2017 28116589

Robjant K, Roberts J, Katona C: Treating posttraumatic stress disorder in female victims of trafficking using narrative exposure therapy: a retrospective audit. Front Psychiatry 8:63, 2017 28620321

Salami T, Gordon M, Coverdale J, et al: What therapies are favored in the treatment of the psychological sequelae of trauma in human trafficking victims. J Psychiatr Pract 24(2):87–96, 2018 29509178

Solomon AL: In search of a job: criminal records as barriers to employment. National Institute of Justice 270:42–51, 2012

Sukach T, Gonzalez N, Cravens Pickens J: Experiences of female sex trafficking survivors: a phenomenological analysis. Qual Rep 23(6):1422–1440, 2018

Surtees R: Monitoring Anti-Trafficking Re/Integration Programmes: A Manual. Brussels, Belgium, King Baudouin Foundation, 2010

Surtees R: Re/Integration of Trafficked Persons: Supporting Economic Empowerment. Vienna, Austria, Nexus Institute, 2012

Thompson J, Haley M: Human trafficking: preparing counselors to work with survivors. International Journal for the Advancement of Counselling 40(3):1–12, 2018

Todd M: Few victims of human trafficking seek visas: most people unaware of T-Visa's protections, attorneys say. News Bank, 2017. Available at: https://infoweb.newsbank.com/apps/news/document-view?p=WORLDNEWSanddocref=news/16855879B572D0C8. Accessed November 6, 2019.

United Nations Office of Drugs and Crime: What is human trafficking? 2014. Available at: www.unodc.org/unodc/en/human-trafficking/what-is-human-trafficking.html. Accessed November 6, 2019.

U.S. Department of Health and Human Services: Screening tool for victims of human trafficking. 2019. Available at: www.acf.hhs.gov/sites/default/files/orr/screening_questions_to_assess_whether_a_person_is_a_trafficking_victim_0.pdf. Accessed November 6, 2019.

Vanwesenbeeck I: Sex work criminalization is barking up the wrong tree. Arch Sex Behav 46(6):1631–1640, 2017 28585156

Weitzer R: Resistance to sex work stigma. Sexualities 21(5–6):717–729, 2018

Wirsing EK: Outreach, collaboration and services to survivors of human trafficking: the Salvation Army STOP-IT program's work in Chicago, Illinois. Social Work and Christianity 39(4):466–480, 2012

Yakushko O: Human trafficking: a review for mental health professionals. International Journal for the Advancement of Counselling 31(3):158–167, 2009

Zimmerman C, Pocock N: Human trafficking and mental health: "my wounds are inside; they are not visible." Brown Journal of World Affairs 19(2):265–280, 2013

Child Sex and Labor Trafficking

Jordan Greenbaum, M.D.

A 15-year-old adolescent runs away from home to escape his father's emotional and physical abuse. After a few days he finds himself without food, shelter, or money. He makes the decision to do what other runaway youth around him are doing: exchange sex for the things he needs.

A 12-year-old Indian girl lives in a very poor village 2 hours from Mumbai. Her parents send her to the city to work as a domestic servant in the home of a wealthy family. She is forced to work 16 hours per day, not allowed to go to school, given minimal food, and is raped by the man in the home.

Trafficking and exploitation of children for labor and/or sex violate the human rights of vulnerable children around the world (United Nations Human Rights and Office of the High Commissioner for Human Rights 1990; U.S. Department of State 2018). The Palermo protocol adopted by the United Nations defines "trafficking in persons" as

> [a] the recruitment, transportation, transfer, harbouring or receipt of persons, by means of the threat or use of force or other forms of coercion, of abduction, of fraud, of deception, of the abuse of power or of a position of vulnerability or of the giving or receiving of payments or benefits to achieve the consent of a person having control over another person, for the purpose of exploitation. Exploitation shall include, at a minimum, the exploitation of the prostitution of others or other forms of sexual exploitation, forced labour or services, slavery or practices similar to slavery, servitude or the removal of organs;

...(c) The recruitment, transportation, transfer, harbouring or receipt of a child for the purpose of exploitation shall be considered "trafficking in persons" even if this does not involve any of the means set forth in subparagraph (a) of this article;... (United Nations Human Rights and Office of the High Commissioner for Human Rights 2000)

Child sexual exploitation may include prostitution, performance in sex-oriented businesses or live web-streamed sex acts, production of child sexual abuse images (formerly called "child pornography"), and forced marriage (Institute of Medicine and National Research Council 2013).

Forced child labor—"work performed by a child under coercion applied by a third party (other than his or her parents) either to the child or to the child's parents, or work performed by a child as a direct consequence of his or her parent or parents being engaged in forced labor" (International Labour Organization 2017, p. 16)—and labor trafficking may occur in agriculture, construction, commercial fishing, manufacturing, domestic servitude, hospitality services, mining, and other sectors or may involve forced begging and engagement in illegal activities (e.g., forced drug smuggling) or door-to-door sales (Buller et al. 2015; United Nations Office on Drugs and Crime 2016; U.S. Department of State 2018). Child trafficking may occur in massage parlors, nail salons, hotels, restaurants, care facilities, and brick kilns; it may be found in war zones, where child soldiers act as scouts, executioners, suicide bombers, and human shields.[1]

Although the United Nations Palermo protocol provides the above definition of human trafficking to guide signatory countries as they create their national anti-trafficking laws (United Nations Human Rights and Office of the High Commissioner for Human Rights 2000), countries vary in their interpretation of the definition, so that a child may be considered "trafficked" in one country and "exploited but not trafficked" in another. Differences are also noted in the specific caveat for children. The Palermo protocol states that force, fraud, coercion and other "means" are not required for sex or labor trafficking involving those less than 18 years of age (United Nations Human

---

[1]"Child" and "children" refer to any person or persons under the age of 18 years. The term *victim* is used in this chapter in its objective, legal sense, indicating a person who has been harmed as a result of some event or action or who has suffered because of someone else's actions. It does not refer to how the person may feel or perceive himself or herself as a result of the event(s) and is not intended to be used to label that person.

Rights and Office of the High Commissioner for Human Rights 2000). U.S. federal law exempts children from the requirement of force, fraud, or coercion *only* for sex trafficking (Trafficking Victims Protection Act of 2000; P.L. 106-386).

The exclusion of "means" from the definition of sex trafficking has major implications: by law, those less than 18 years of age cannot legally consent to commercial sexual exploitation. Therefore, children who exchange sexual acts for items of value of any kind are considered victims of child sex trafficking (CST), even if they report "consenting" to the process and initiating the activities themselves (e.g., posting an ad on social media). This is demonstrated in the first case example, above. This exclusion of means from the definition allows many more children to access important social services. Because of mandated reporting laws, however, it also carries the potential unintended consequence of causing runaway/homeless children to avoid needed medical care because of fears that health professionals will report them to authorities.

EPIDEMIOLOGY

Acknowledging that estimates of the prevalence of human trafficking are fraught with difficulties as outlined in previous chapters, the International Labour Organization has estimated that approximately 4.5 million of the world's children are involved in forced labor (of which, approximately 1 million have experienced commercial sexual exploitation), and 5.7 million are victims of forced marriage (International Labour Organization 2017). Reliable statistics for child trafficking are lacking in the United States, although research on runaway/homeless youth and young adults demonstrates high rates of "survival sex," ranging from 10% to 50% (Chettiar et al. 2010; Greene et al. 1999; Walls and Bell 2011). In a recent study involving 641 youth receiving services at Covenant House sites in the United States and Canada, the total prevalence of trafficking was 19% (14% sex trafficking, 8% labor trafficking, and 3% both sex and labor) (Murphy 2016).

There may be differences in demographics between persons identified as having been subjected to labor versus sex trafficking in the United States. Of confirmed cases of adult and child sex trafficking, identified in the U.S. Human Trafficking Reporting System between January 2008 and June 2010, 83% were U.S. citizens/U.S. nationals and 94% were female. In contrast, of confirmed labor trafficking victims, less than 2% were U.S. citizens/U.S. nationals and 68% were female (Banks and Kyckelhahn 2011). However, extreme caution should be used in interpreting these statistics as they reflect only *identified* victims and are subject to biases associated with recognition and reporting. It is likely that statistics are influenced by cultural beliefs about gender (males are protectors not victims), lack of awareness that boys and transgender youth are sexually exploited, prioritization in investigation (sex trafficking over labor trafficking), misidentification (foreign nationals viewed as illegal immigrants and deported rather than trafficking victims needing services), and difficulty in detection and recognition of exploitation (Hohendorff et al. 2017).

As noted in Table 11–1, factors creating vulnerability to human trafficking may be found at the individual, relationship, community, and societal levels (Acharya et al. 2018; Cole 2018; Landers et al. 2017; Ottisova et al. 2016; Perry and McEwing 2013; Reid 2018; Self-Brown et al. 2018). Globally, children living on the streets are at increased risk of trafficking/exploitation (Davis et al. 2016; Murphy 2016; Walls and Bell 2011). In many cases, they have run away from home to escape family dysfunction in the form of intrafamilial violence, sexual abuse, caregiver substance misuse, or parental intolerance of their gay/lesbian/bisexual/transgender status (Dank et al. 2015; McIntyre 2009; Reid et al. 2017; Silverman et al. 2007a; Wolfe et al. 2018). Child maltreatment is a major risk factor: in a study of sex-trafficked children receiving treatment for serious behavioral health issues, nearly 87% reported a history of sexual abuse and 58% reported moderate to severe neglect (Landers et al. 2017). Those with substance abuse disorders are at increased risk of trafficking, especially youth using intravenous drugs (Kerr et al. 2009). Communities of marginalized families and those in impoverished circumstances are at risk (Hepburn and Simon 2013; U.S. Department of State 2018), as are children who live in areas frequented by tourists and business travelers (Klain 1999).

Extreme poverty and forced migration are powerful social determinants of child trafficking (Gozdziak and Bump 2008; Hepburn and Simon 2013; International Centre for Migration Policy Development 2015; Perry and McEwing 2013; UNICEF 2017; United Nations High Commissioner for Refugees 2014). Poverty and unemployment may cause families to send their children to large cities to seek work, thereby rendering the children vulnerable to exploitation and trafficking. Migrating children fleeing community violence, armed conflict, or other social disruption may travel alone or may become separated from family during the journey. Their lack of adult care

TABLE 11–1. Vulnerability factors for child trafficking

INDIVIDUAL	RELATIONSHIP	COMMUNITY	SOCIETAL
Sexual/physical/emotional abuse and/or neglect	Intrafamilial violence	Natural disaster	Bias/discrimination against females
Runaway/homelessness	Bullying/ostracism	Tolerance of violence, commercial sex	Rigid roles for males (discourage disclosure)
Substance misuse	Parental substance misuse	Widespread poverty and limited employment opportunities	Homophobia and intolerance of alternative sexual identities/ orientation
Untreated mental health problems	Gang affiliation		
	Familial poverty	Limited parental knowledge of trafficking	Marginalization of certain populations
Cognitive delay/learning disability	Family involvement in criminal activities		
	Limited education	Mass migration	Limited rights of children
Involvement with child protective services and/or juvenile justice system	Familial roles discriminating against females/children	Increased tourism and business travelers	Widespread social upheaval/ corruption
Difficulties in school	Limited knowledge of trafficking	Organized crime in area	Cultural beliefs/stigma
Risky internet behavior		Drug use, sales	Lack of policy or weak enforcement of anti-trafficking laws
LGBTQ status	Limited maternal education	Corruption of local officials	
Lack of identity and/or immigration documents			Insecure borders

Note. LGBTQ=Lesbian/gay/bisexual/transgender/queer/questioning.

and support, lack of identification documents (e.g., birth certificates, passports), their young age and limited job skills, and their lack of knowledge of the host country language, culture, and laws make them extremely vulnerable to labor and sex trafficking/exploitation (International Centre for Migration Policy Development 2015; United Nations High Commissioner for Refugees 2014).

Children living in communities affected by natural disasters, such as the earthquake and tsunami in Indonesia in 2018, may find themselves orphaned, homeless, and without any means of support. They are vulnerable to traffickers who may move into the area to seek cheap labor and persons to sell into the sex trade. Finally, cultural beliefs and practices influence vulnerability to human trafficking at the societal level (Chung 2009; Gjermeni et al. 2008; Perry and McEwing 2013), with gender bias/violence, the belief that children are the property of parents, and discrimination against certain social/racial/ethnic/religious/socioeconomic or other groups playing major roles.

Children may be recruited into trafficking/exploitation by parents, other relatives, intimate partners, acquaintances, peers, respected members of the local community, employers, or strangers (Cole 2018; Hornor and Sherfield 2018; Moore et al. 2017; Reid 2016; Wolfe et al. 2018). Common recruitment methods in the United States and around the world include false romances and seduction (especially males seducing females); false promises of money, jobs, or a "better life"; violence and force (e.g., recruitment by gangs) and/or kidnapping (with or without use of drugs); "bait and switch" methods; and relationships formed on the internet (Acharya et al. 2018; Baldwin et al. 2011; Moore et al. 2017; Polaris 2016; Reid 2016; Silverman et al. 2007a).

> A 16-year-old adolescent who lived in a village near Tijuana, Mexico, was befriended by a 25-year-old man during a community event. She became romantically involved with him, and he promised her and her family that he would marry her when they traveled to the United States for a "better life." On arrival in the United States, he took her to a cantina where she was forced to serve drinks and provide sex to 10–15 clients per night.

HEALTH NEEDS OF TRAFFICKED CHILDREN

Globally, labor- and sex-trafficked children are at increased risk for numerous medical and mental health problems, including sexually transmitted infections, HIV/AIDS, unwanted pregnancy and associated complications, substance misuse, traumatic and work-related injury, malnutrition, dehydration, chronic pain, PTSD and complex PTSD symptoms, depression and suicidality, oppositional defiant disorder and other behavioral problems, somatic symptoms, and anxiety disorders (Acharya et al. 2018; Frey et al. 2018; Hornor and Sherfield 2018; Le et al. 2018; Omole 2016; Ottisova et al. 2018a, 2018b; Silverman et al. 2007a; Sprang and Cole 2018). In a study of Nepalese girls and women sex trafficked in India, 60.6% of those less than 15 years old tested positive for HIV (Silverman et al. 2007b). In one study of sex-trafficked adolescents in the United States, 78% met DSM-IV criteria for PTSD and 50% had attempted suicide in the prior year (Edinburgh et al. 2015). In another U.S. study of sex-trafficked youth, 92% reported using/misusing drugs or alcohol (Moore et al. 2017). Drug/alcohol misuse may predate the onset of trafficking and serve as a "push" factor for exploitation but may also occur during the period of exploitation in efforts to ease stress or physical pain or to stay awake for many hours. In some cases, trafficked children are expected to drink alcohol or use drugs with the clients, and they may be given substances by the trafficker (Acharya et al. 2018; Polaris 2016).

Studies of labor and sex trafficking from across the globe consistently document trauma occurring during the trafficking experience, often in the form of violence, threats, deplorable living conditions, stigma, and discrimination (Davis and Miles 2018; Ottisova et al. 2016; Sprang and Cole 2018). In one study of children involved in intrafamilial sex trafficking, 58.1% experienced physical assault, and 25.7% sustained bruising, fractures, or cuts while being trafficked (Sprang and Cole 2018). In another study of male and female youth receiving posttrafficking services, severe physical violence was associated with depression (adjusted odds ratio [AOR], 3.55), anxiety (AOR, 2.13), and suicidal ideation (AOR, 3.68; 95% CI, 1.77–7.67) (Kiss et al. 2015). Sexual violence experienced during trafficking was associated with depression (AOR, 2.27) and suicidal ideation (AOR, 3.43).

Work-related trauma and illness associated with labor trafficking vary with the occupation but can be severe or even fatal (U.S. Department of State 2018). For example, adults and children trafficked in the fishing industry may drown after being dragged overboard by a net or getting entangled in underwater nets. They may suffer from exposure to extreme cold or heat, sustain injuries from fishing hooks, fish bites, or unguarded machinery; they may suffer from exhaustion and malnutrition (Hamenoo and Sottie 2015; Pocock et al. 2018). In one study of labor-trafficked men and boys in the Greater Mekong Subregion (predominantly involving fishing, manufacturing, and begging), 35.5% had sustained a work-related injury and nearly 30% received no personal protective equipment (Pocock et al. 2016).

Many trafficked children experience early childhood trauma (Cook et al. 2018), sometimes chronic in nature, and these early traumatic experiences may contribute to some of the long-term consequences associated with human trafficking. Repetitive and/or chronic trauma in the lives of trafficked children before and during their exploitation may help explain why some demonstrate symptoms of complex PTSD (defined by the ICD-11 task force as the presence of the core symptoms of PTSD, plus problems with affect dysregulation, negative self-concept, and relational difficulties) (Maercker et al. 2013; Ottisova et al. 2018a). In a study of labor and sex-trafficked children with PTSD, Ottisova et al. (2018a) documented alterations in affect regulation (82%), self-perception (64%), relationships (54%), and somatization (64%).

BARRIERS AND CHALLENGES TO HEALTH CARE ACCESS AND ENGAGEMENT

In the United States, there is evidence that sex-trafficked children frequently have contact with medical and mental health professionals during and surrounding the time they are exploited (Goldberg et al. 2017; Sprang and Cole 2018; Varma et al. 2015). In one study of intrafamilial sex trafficking, 51.6% of children had been in contact with health care professionals and 54.9% with community mental health providers (Sprang and Cole 2018). In another study of trafficked youth receiving services at an emergency department or child advocacy center, 93.6% had a history of a mental health disorder, and nearly 40% had been in contact with behavioral health services (Hornor and Sherfield 2018).

Although access to medical and mental health care may be feasible for sex-trafficked children in parts of the United States, much less is known about access to health care by those who are trafficked for labor. In addition, access to formal health care may be quite limited in other countries (Pocock et al. 2018). Even in high-resource countries, numerous barriers to care may exist (Albright et al. 2020), such as availability of qualified, trained providers, accessibility to clinics and hospitals, acceptability of the quality of care offered by professionals, affordability of care, and accommodation of service providers to the needs of trafficked persons (see Table 11–2). Although mental health professionals cannot easily modify certain barriers (e.g., location of clinic, Medicaid reimbursement, paucity of interpreters), they may address other barriers through simple environmental alterations (e.g., making waiting room child friendly, posting signage in multiple languages) and training and education of staff.

Training on human trafficking and trauma-informed principles of care is limited in the United States and other countries (Beck et al. 2015; Macias-Konstantopoulos et al. 2015; Ross et al. 2015; Viergever et al. 2015), and trafficked persons have reported feeling shamed, blamed, and stigmatized by health care professionals (Ijadi-Maghsoodi et al. 2018; Rajaram and Tidball 2018). A failure to practice a patient-centered, culturally sensitive, trauma-informed, and rights-based approach may drive many victims to avoid mental health and medical services (Rajaram and Tidball 2018). In many regions there is a paucity of mental health professionals formally trained in trauma-focused therapy or other relevant forms of mental health treatment and limited experience with complex trauma (Macias-Konstantopoulos et al. 2015). Providers may lack experience treating children or those identifying as LGBTQ. All these limitations negatively impact accessibility and acceptability of health care (West Coast Children's Clinic et al. 2018).

Accommodation is an important factor in health care access; to serve trafficked children, one needs to consider their circumstances. They may be living on the streets and seek care late at night; they may live with a trafficker who does not allow them to seek care or live with parents or foster parents who work in daytime or night jobs. Trafficked children and parents with limited resources may have difficulty committing to and following through on an appointment for a future date. Children involved in the child protection system may experience frequent moves related to foster care; many trafficked youths continue to run away periodically and may be lost to follow-up for an extended period. Flexibility in clinic hours, the availability of walk-in appointments, and a policy of not dismissing patients from a practice because of "no-shows" help address these issues, as does the ability to deliver mental health therapy in the community rather than in a fixed office or hospital (Judge et al. 2018; West Coast Children's Clinic et al. 2018).

Once a trafficked child has been connected with services, there are many factors that can complicate treatment. Inherent characteristics of trafficking (e.g., coercion, control, unpredictability, abusive

TABLE 11–2. Potential barriers to medical and mental health care access and engagement

AVAILABILITY	ACCESSIBILITY	ACCEPTABILITY	AFFORDABILITY	ACCOMMODATION
Inadequate numbers of providers or interpreters available	Facility located far from patient	Providers lack training in human trafficking, TIC, rights-based care	Lack of free care	Limited hours of operation
Limited or no ability to respond to patient preference for gender of provider	Facility not near public transportation	Providers lack training in trauma-focused mental health treatment strategies and other appropriate types of treatment	Sliding scale not helpful	No walk-in appointments
	Citizenship requirements		Demand for up-front payment for services	Long wait time after arrival
Lack of available assessment tools, private rooms, and medications	Victim status requirements	Providers do not demonstrate cultural sensitivity (e.g., do not respect beliefs, cultural practices regarding healing)	Costly medications	Long wait time to schedule appointments
			Limited access to free mental health services (e.g., visit limits)	Low tolerance of no-show and late appointments
Lack of adequate referral system for advanced mental health and nonhealth services (e.g., immigration, legal, housing)		No facility protocol to guide response to suspected trafficking		Lack of flexibility in responding to patient needs off-hours
		Environment is not child friendly		
		Staff lack training in pediatric care		
Lack of addiction treatment centers		Staff lack training in care for LGBTQ youth		
Poor interagency and provider communication and lack of comprehensive case management		Lack of patient information (especially in native language)		

Note. TIC=trauma-informed care.

relationships), ongoing involvement in trafficking, as well as symptoms of complex trauma, may render mental health engagement and
treatment of CST youth especially challenging (Cohen et al. 2017;
Judge et al. 2018). It may be difficult for trafficked children to trust
adult care providers, experience a sense of agency that allows them
to actively participate in treatment planning, or commit to regular
visits over an extended period (West Coast Children's Clinic et al.
2018). Concerns about legal issues (criminal charges the child may
face related, or unrelated, to their trafficking experience) and immigration problems may exacerbate traumatic stress symptoms and
make it difficult for clients to engage in mental health treatment.
Coexisting substance use disorders or preexisting mental health
problems complicate treatment. Avoidance, dissociation, affect dysregulation, and problems with interpersonal relationships may impact client engagement and the course of therapy (Judge et al. 2018;
West Coast Children's Clinic et al. 2018). Because of trauma bonding
with a trafficker, intrafamilial trafficking, normalization of exploitation in the child's life, lack of awareness of labor laws and rights, or
the need to feel in control of one's life, a child may not perceive themselves as having been exploited or in need of treatment (Cohen et al.
2017; Greenbaum et al. 2015).

In one study of trafficked youth receiving services, 49.2% were
not aware of their exploitation, and 68% showed evidence of trauma
bonding. In a study of foreign national survivors of trafficking, Gozdziak and Bump (2008) found that many of the children viewed
their exploitation as "work." Because this work was often facilitated
by family members, they did not perceive the situation as exploitative. Instead, they felt they were helping the family earn money.

Finally, cultural differences between provider and client may complicate engagement in mental health services. Working with clients
from a different culture requires sensitivity, an open mind, and commitment to collaboration (Bryant and Njenga 2006; Rafferty 2017).
As demonstrated in the Gozdziak and Bump (2008) study, different
cultural views about the responsibilities of children to work and financially contribute to the family may lead to vastly different inter-
pretations of a child's work situation (labor trafficking by parent vs.
contributing to family welfare, with assistance of parent). Differences in cultural views about gender, social hierarchies, the role of
the child in a family, the importance of the individual compared with
the collective group (family or community), the role of fate versus individual agency, and the importance of past versus future will all impact the way mental health professionals and their clients perceive

the trafficking situation and how best to treat symptoms (Rafferty 2017). The Western focus on the individual, on "talking therapy," and the need to identify and process emotions and cognitions may make treatment very difficult for trafficked children from other cultures (Chung 2009), and some service providers feel that Western therapy is not always appropriate for treatment (Rafferty 2017). The fact that some languages lack words for certain emotions has implications for the way the emotional mind is viewed in that society. Symptoms of depression, anxiety, or PTSD may be attributed to physical problems, and clients may seek medical treatment rather than mental health resources (Rafferty 2017). A culture's views of psychopathology may prohibit a child from acknowledging emotional distress; the cultural views on sex may prohibit any discussion of the topic, much less forced/coerced sex and commercial sex.

Not only do religious and cultural beliefs influence engagement in mental health therapy, they also may impact recovery, facilitating resilience from trauma (Chung 2009) or exerting harmful influences. On the one hand, spirituality can help a victim find meaning in their experiences and feel a sense of hope. On the other hand, corruption of religious and cultural beliefs can effectively bind victims to their exploitative situation and make treatment difficult. An example of the latter may be found in the use of juju practices by human traffickers. A firm belief in the power of the supernatural permeates Nigerian culture, and traffickers have used juju practices to manipulate and control their victims. A juju ceremony begins with a traditional priest performing prescribed religious activities, after which a person solemnly swears to fulfill a promise (in the case of trafficking, the victim promises to "obey" the trafficker, pay back their debt, and never disclose the trafficker's identity). The person believes that should he or she break that promise, he or she and his or her family will be brought to harm and destruction by the gods. Nigerian trafficking victims who have experienced the juju ceremony comply with their traffickers' demands out of tremendous fear (van der Watt and Kruger 2017). Presumably, subsequent mental health therapy may be quite difficult, especially if the meaning and impact of this cultural practice were ignored by the practitioner.

MENTAL HEALTH THERAPY FOR TRAFFICKED CHILDREN

Currently, a solid evidence base for mental health treatment of trafficked children is lacking (Judge 2018; Judge et al. 2018; Salami et al. 2018; West Coast Children's Clinic et al. 2018). The West Coast Children's Clinic developed the C-Change program specifically for sexually exploited youth (West Coast Children's Clinic et al. 2018). This treatment modality uses concepts from attachment theory, psychodynamic theory, and multiple modalities designed for complex trauma treatment. Studies of the effectiveness of this therapy modality have not been published. Other efforts to treat CST involve modifications of therapeutic strategies designed for complex trauma, sexual abuse, interpersonal violence, and torture. With few exceptions, outcome studies of these modified strategies are yet to be published (O'Callaghan et al. 2013; West Coast Children's Clinic et al. 2018). O'Callaghan and colleagues used group-based, culturally modified, and trauma-focused cognitive-behavioral therapy to treat sexually exploited, war-affected females in the Democratic Republic of Congo. They demonstrated significant decreases in trauma symptoms and improvement in symptoms of depression, anxiety, conduct problems, and prosocial behavior (O'Callaghan et al. 2013). Other therapeutic strategies for CST treatment include modifications of dialectical behavior therapy, Trauma Affect Regulation: Guide for Education and Therapy (TARGET), and integrated treatment for complex trauma (West Coast Children's Clinic et al. 2018). Therapeutic strategies that do not conform to the traditional Western "talk therapies" are beginning to be studied formally, as in the Sampoornata (fulfillment) dance/movement therapy used by Kolkata Sanved with survivors of trafficking (Fargnoli 2017).

Traditional healers in some cultures may be able to provide considerable relief to traumatized children. Chung (2009) relates an instance in which cooperation between the psychologist and Buddhist monks led to the healing of Asian rape victims, families, and the community:

> To more effectively address the psychological pain associated with the rapes and abuse, I simultaneously worked with a Buddhist monk to develop a cleansing ritual for the girls. The rape and sexual abuse were extremely difficult topics to discuss given the associated cultural stigma and shame. Some of the girls talked about not being accepted into their communities as a result of being raped...everyone knew about the rape and sexual abuse, but it was a taboo subject and therefore no one discussed it. Given their strong spiritual beliefs, I made contact with a Buddhist monk and inquired about creating a Buddhist cleansing ritual for the rape survivors. The cleansing ritual performed by the monks proved to be a powerful healing mechanism not only for individuals, but also for their families and communities. (p. 92)

This example demonstrates the importance of mental health professionals and other service providers making every effort to understand the cultural beliefs and practices relevant to their trafficked clients and families, to be sensitive to the issues impacting how people interpret traumatic experiences and how they may best recover (Rafferty 2017; Rechtman 2000). Professionals need to be willing to collaborate with respected indigenous healers when doing so will not harm a child and may well help with the healing process (Chung 2009; Gozdziak and Bump 2008) Incorporating cultural practices into Western therapies may also be helpful, as in using meditation, mindfulness, yoga, or tai chi chuan (Bryant and Njenga 2006). There is a great need for research on the effectiveness of Western and non-Western treatment modalities with sex- and labor-trafficked children. It is likely that combinations of therapeutic approaches, with flexibility in tailoring treatment to the individual's needs and cultural beliefs, will prove most successful.

As work continues in the effort to develop effective mental health treatment strategies for trafficked adults and children, several recommendations have been made, based on research with survivors and treatment providers (see Table 11–3) (Chung 2009; Gordon et al. 2018; Ijadi-Maghsoodi et al. 2018; Judge et al. 2018; Powell et al. 2018; Rafferty 2017; Rajaram and Tidball 2018; Recknor et al. 2018; Salami et al. 2018; Steiner et al. 2018; West Coast Children's Clinic et al. 2018).

CONCLUSION

Globally, children who are trafficked for sex and/or labor typically have multiple factors placing them at risk for exploitation. Many of these factors involve traumatic experiences and deprivation. They experience additional trauma during their period of exploitation, ranging from violence and traumatic injury to illness, from threats to self and family to debt bondage, from deprivation of food and sleep to forced drug/alcohol use. Many survivors of trafficking emerge with significant mental health issues and symptoms of complex trauma. Although research has not yet provided an evidence base to guide mental health providers in their efforts to treat trauma symptoms, efforts are being made to modify other evidence-based therapies, tailoring interventions to meet the diverse needs of trafficked children. A successful intervention must include an awareness of, and respect for, how culture impacts human trafficking and consideration of the inherent characteristics of human trafficking that make mental health intervention particularly challenging.

TABLE 11-3. Recommendations for mental health care of trafficked persons

Service delivery

- Incorporate mental health services into primary care and reproductive health practices (co-located services).

- Consider alternative methods of service delivery to increase access (e.g., mobile clinics).

- Consider providing services in nontraditional settings within the community (e.g., park, car, restaurant).

- Create system in which clients can contact mental health professionals urgently.

- Adopt flexible rescheduling practices to accommodate interruptions in treatment (avoid closing a case because of no-shows).

- Encourage engagement by frequent telephone calls/text messages to client.

Collaboration

- Know details of services provided by referral agencies, and contact agency directly when making a referral ("warm hand-off").

- Assign a case manager to facilitate cross-agency collaboration and service delivery.

- Prioritize multidisciplinary collaboration that includes mental health (e.g., care teams); engage in cross-training of multidisciplinary team members to clarify role of mental health in recovery and reintegration.

- Assess psychosocial needs and provide services or refer for services (e.g., housing, work skills training, immigration issues).

Workforce

- Increase workforce of qualified mental health providers through training and hiring:

  - Include training on human trafficking, trauma-informed care, and complex trauma.

  - Ensure adequate supervision of practitioners.

  - Ensure staff are culturally competent.

- Increase number of, and access to, trained interpreters.

- Educate mental health professionals on secondary traumatic stress and incorporate methods. of addressing secondary traumatic stress in facility policies and practices.

TABLE 11–3.   Recommendations for mental health care of trafficked persons *(continued)*

Therapeutic approaches

- Tailor all aspects of mental health therapy to meet the needs and circumstances of the trafficked person (type and process of therapy, meeting place, meeting time, engagement steps, definition of treatment success, cultural values, and beliefs).

- Maintain consistency and predictability in care providers.

- Prioritize treatment of coexisting substance misuse disorders.

- Use trauma-informed principles:

  - Use nonjudgmental, empathic, respectful approach.

  - Ensure absence of bias/discrimination/stigma related to gender/sexual orientation/age/religion/ ethnicity/race/citizenship/culture.

  - Ensure confidentiality and privacy.

  - Support self-determination and encourage participation in decision-making.

- Understand that client may continue to be trafficked or otherwise traumatized during time frame of counseling.

- Address physical and psychological safety, and work with client to establish safety plan (important throughout therapy).

- Provide psychoeducation to the trafficked person about trauma, traumatic stress responses, and behavioral adaptations to hostile, dangerous, and unpredictable circumstances.

- Empower client to build social support system and access services.

- View client's circumstances through a social justice lens to understand the influence of social, political, and economic factors.

- Provide psychological support and psychoeducation for trafficked persons' family members and others in support system.

- Respect cultural and religious beliefs and practices as well as gender identity and sexual orientation.

- Ensure practices are culturally relevant and sensitive.

- As indicated, consider use of alternative methods of treatment that integrate traditional healing processes and holistic healing strategies and incorporate cultural traditions and beliefs into therapy.

- Consider nonverbal therapeutic activities such as dance/movement therapy or music therapy as indicated.

- Consider pharmacologic therapy, as appropriate, to supplement other forms of therapy, and to be directed by a psychiatrist trained in trauma.

Pearls and Pointers

- Vulnerability factors for labor or sex trafficking occur at the individual, relationship, community, and societal levels.

- Myriad health and mental health problems are associated with child trafficking, some of which may be debilitating or even fatal.

- Trafficked children often experience high levels of depressive and posttraumatic stress symptoms, as well as symptoms of complex trauma.

- An evidence base to guide mental health practitioners on treating trafficked children is lacking, and many professionals are using modified versions of evidence-based therapies designed for child sexual abuse, intimate partner violence, or torture.

- Recommendations for mental health professionals include the need for sensitivity with respect to culture, race/ethnicity, spirituality, gender, and sexual orientation.

- Globally, a variety of mental health treatment strategies are being used, including Western "talk therapies," and nonverbal therapeutic modalities such as dance/movement therapy, art and music therapy, yoga, and meditation. In some cases, modalities are being combined, incorporating some aspects of nonverbal modalities with cognitive therapeutic approaches.

REFERENCES

Acharya AK, Sotelo LSP, Nino JJC: The harmful sexual and nonsexual behaviors of trafficked women and children in Mexico: a study of victims of sexual exploitation. Dignity 3(2):3, 2018

Albright K, Greenbaum J, Edwards S, Tsai C: Systematic review of facilitators of, barriers to, and recommendations for healthcare services for child survivors of human trafficking globally. Child Abuse Neglect 100:104289, Feb 2020 31787336

Baldwin SB, Eisenman DP, Sayles JN, et al: Identification of human trafficking victims in health care settings. Health Hum Rights 13(1):E36–E49, 2011 22772961

Banks D, Kyckelhahn T: Characteristics of suspected human trafficking incidents, 2008–2010. United States Department of Justice, April 2011. Available at: www.bjs.gov/content/pub/pdf/cshti0810.pdf. Accessed November 6, 2019.

Beck ME, Lineer MM, Melzer-Lange M, et al: Medical providers' understanding of sex trafficking and their experience with at-risk patients. Pediatrics 135(4):e895–e902, 2015 25780076

Bryant RA, Njenga FG: Cultural sensitivity: making trauma assessment and treatment plans culturally relevant. J Clin Psychiatry 67(Suppl 2):74–79, 2006 16602819

Buller AM, Vaca V, Stoklosa H, et al: Labour exploitation, trafficking and migrant health: multi-country findings on the health risks and consequences of migrant and trafficked workers. International Organization for Migration and London School of Hygiene and Tropical Medicine, 2015. Available at: https://publications.iom.int/system/files/pdf/labour_exploitation_trafficking_en.pdf. Accessed November 6, 2019.

Chettiar J, Shannon K, Wood E, et al: Survival sex work involvement among street-involved youth who use drugs in a Canadian setting. J Public Health (Oxf) 32(3):322–327, 2010 20061578

Chung RCY: Cultural perspectives on child trafficking, human rights and social justice: a model for psychologists. Counselling Psychological Quarterly 22(1):85–96, 2009

Cohen JA, Mannarino AP, Kinnish K: Trauma-focused cognitive behavioral therapy for commercially sexually exploited youth. J Child Adolesc Trauma 10(2):175–185, 2017 28690714

Cole J: Service providers' perspectives on sex trafficking of male minors: comparing background and trafficking situations of male and female victims. Child and Adolescent Social Work Journal 35(4):423–433, 2018

Cook MC, Barnert E, Ijadi-Maghsoodi R, et al: Exploring mental health and substance use treatment needs of commercially sexually exploited youth participating in a specialty juvenile court. Behav Med 44(3):242–249, 2018 29558256

Dank M, Yahner J, Madden K, et al: Surviving the streets of New York: experiences of LGBTQ youth, YMSM, and YWSW engaged in survival sex. Urban Institute, 2015. Available at: www.urban.org/sites/default/files/publication/42186/2000119-Surviving-the-Streets-of-New-York.pdf. Accessed November 6, 2019.

Davis J, Miles G: They chase us like dogs: exploring the vulnerabilities of "ladyboys" in the Cambodian sex trade. Dignity 3(2), 2018

Davis J, Fiss J, Miles G: "To help my parents…": An exploratory study on the hidden vulnerabilities of street-involved children and youth in Chiang Mai, Thailand. February 2016. Available at: www.academia.edu/25039251/To_Help_My_Parents. Accessed November 6, 2019.

Edinburgh L, Pape-Blabolil J, Harpin SB, et al: Assessing exploitation experiences of girls and boys seen at a child advocacy center. Child Abuse Negl 46:47–59, 2015 25982287

Fargnoli A: Maintaining stability in the face of adversity: self-care practices of human trafficking survivor-trainers in India. American Journal of Dance Therapy 39(2):226–251, 2017

Frey LM, Middleton J, Gattis MN, et al: Suicidal ideation and behavior among youth victims of sex trafficking in Kentuckiana. Crisis 40(4):240–248, 2018 30375247

Gjermeni E, Van Hook MP, Gjipali S, et al: Trafficking of children in Albania: patterns of recruitment and reintegration. Child Abuse Negl 32(10):941–948, 2008 18995900

Goldberg AP, Moore JL, Houck C, et al: Domestic minor sex trafficking patients: a retrospective analysis of medical presentation. J Pediatr Adolesc Gynecol 30(1):109–115, 2017 27575407

Gordon M, Salami T, Coverdale J, et al: Psychiatry's role in the management of human trafficking victims: an integrated care approach. J Psychiatr Pract 24(2):79–86, 2018 29509177

Gozdziak E, Bump MN: Victims no longer: research on child survivors of trafficking for sexual and labor exploitation in the United States. U.S. Department of Justice Report (Doc No 221891), March 2008. Available at: www.ncjrs.gov/pdffiles1/nij/grants/221891.pdf. Accessed November 6, 2019.

Greenbaum J, Crawford-Jakubiak JE; Committee on Child Abuse and Neglect: Child sex trafficking and commercial sexual exploitation: health care needs of victims. Pediatrics 135(3):566–574, 2015 25713283

Greene JM, Ennett ST, Ringwalt CL: Prevalence and correlates of survival sex among runaway and homeless youth. Am J Public Health 89(9):1406–1409, 1999 10474560

Hamenoo ES, Sottie CA: Stories from Lake Volta: the lived experiences of trafficked children in Ghana. Child Abuse Negl 40:103–112, 2015 25015268

Hepburn S, Simon RJ: Human Trafficking Around the World: Hidden in Plain Sight. New York, Columbia University Press, 2013

Hohendorff JV, Habigzang LF, Koller SH: "A boy, being a victim, nobody really buys that, you know?": Dynamics of sexual violence against boys. Child Abuse Negl 70:53–64, 2017 28558323

Hornor G, Sherfield J: Commercial sexual exploitation of children: health care use and case characteristics. J Pediatr Health Care 32(3):250–262, 2018 29422230

Ijadi-Maghsoodi R, Bath E, Cook M, et al: Commercially sexually exploited youths' health care experiences, barriers, and recommendations: a qualitative analysis. Child Abuse Negl 76:334–341, 2018 29195171

Institute of Medicine and National Research Council: Confronting Commercial Sexual Exploitation and Sex Trafficking of Minors in the United States. Washington, DC, National Academies Press, 2013

International Centre for Migration Policy Development: Targeting Vulnerabilities: The Impact of the Syrian War and Refugee Situation on Trafficking in Persons: A Study of Syria, Turkey, Lebanon, Jordan, and Iraq. Vienna, Austria, International Centre for Migration Policy Development, 2015

International Labour Organization: Global estimates of modern slavery: forced labour and forced marriage. September 19, 2017. Available at: www.ilo.org/wcmsp5/groups/public/---dgreports/---dcomm/documents/publication/wcms_575479.pdf. Accessed October 23, 2019.

Judge AM: Uncharted waters: developing mental health services for survivors of domestic human sex trafficking. Harv Rev Psychiatry 26(5):287–297, 2018 30188340

Judge AM, Murphy JA, Hidalgo J, et al: Engaging survivors of human trafficking: complex health care needs and scarce resources. Ann Intern Med 168(9):658–663, 2018 29532076

Kerr T, Marshall BDL, Miller C, et al: Injection drug use among street-involved youth in a Canadian setting. BMC Public Health 9:171–177, 2009 19493353

Kiss L, Yun K, Pocock N, Zimmerman C: Exploitation, violence, and suicide risk among child and adolescent survivors of human trafficking in the Greater Mekong subregion. JAMA Pediatr 169:e152278, 2015

Klain E: Prostitution of Children and Child-Sex Tourism: An Analysis of Domestic and International Responses. Alexandria, VA, National Center for Missing and Exploited Children, 1999

Landers M, McGrath K, Johnson MH, et al: Baseline characteristics of dependent youth who have been commercially sexually exploited: findings from a specialized treatment program. J Child Sex Abuse 26(6):692–709, 2017 28656806

Le PD, Ryan N, Rosenstock Y, et al: Health issues associated with commercial sexual exploitation and sex trafficking of children in the United States: a systematic review. Behav Med 44(3):219–233, 2018 30020867

Macias-Konstantopoulos WL, Munroe D, Purcell G, et al: The commercial sexual exploitation and sex trafficking of minors in the Boston metropolitan area: experiences and challenges faced by front-line providers and other stakeholders. Journal of Applied Research on Children 6(1):4, 2015

Maercker A, Brewin CR, Bryant RA, et al: Diagnosis and classification of disorders specifically associated with stress: proposals for ICD-11. World Psychiatry 12(3):198–206, 2013 24096776

McIntyre S: Under the radar: the sexual exploitation of young men—Western Canadian Edition. 2009. Accessed at: http://humanservices.alberta.ca/documents/child-sexual-exploitation-under-the-radar-western-canada.pdf. Accessed November 6, 2019.

Moore JL, Houck C, Hirway P, et al: Trafficking experiences and psychosocial features of domestic minor sex trafficking victims. J Interpers Violence April 1:886260517703373, 2017 29294728

Murphy LT: Labor and sex trafficking among homeless youth: a ten-city study executive summary. 2016. Available at: https://covenanthousestudy.org/landing/trafficking/docs/Loyola-Research-Results.pdf. Accessed November 6, 2019.

O'Callaghan P, McMullen J, Shannon C, et al: A randomized controlled trial of trauma-focused cognitive behavioral therapy for sexually exploited, war-affected Congolese girls. J Am Acad Child Adolesc Psychiatry 52(4):359–369, 2013 23582867

Omole C: Human trafficking: the health of men forced into labor trafficking in the United States. Doctoral dissertation, Walden University, 2016. Available at: https://scholarworks.waldenu.edu/cgi/viewcontent.cgi?article=3083andcontext=dissertations. Accessed November 6, 2019.

Ottisova L, Hemmings S, Howard LM, et al: Prevalence and risk of violence and the mental, physical and sexual health problems associated with human trafficking: an updated systematic review. Epidemiol Psychiatr Sci 25(4):317–341, 2016 27066701

Ottisova L, Smith P, Oram S: Psychological consequences of human trafficking: complex posttraumatic stress disorder in trafficked children. Behav Med 44(3):234–241, 2018a 30020865

Ottisova L, Smith P, Shetty H, et al: Psychological consequences of child trafficking: an historical cohort study of trafficked children in contact with secondary mental health services. PLOS One 13(3):e0192321, 2018b 29518186

Perry KM, McEwing L: How do social determinants affect human trafficking in Southeast Asia, and what can we do about it? A systematic review. Health Hum Rights 15(2):138–159, 2013 24421161

Pocock NS, Kiss L, Oram S, et al: Labour trafficking among men and boys in the greater Mekong subregion: exploitation, violence, occupational health risks and injuries. PLOS One 11(12):e0168500, 2016 27992583

Pocock NS, Nguyen LH, Lucero-Prisno Iii DE, et al: Occupational, physical, sexual and mental health and violence among migrant and trafficked commercial fishers and seafarers from the Greater Mekong Subregion (GMS): systematic review. Glob Health Res Policy 3:28–41, 2018 30288452

Polaris: More than drinks for sale: exposing sex trafficking in cantinas and bars in the U.S. 2016. Available at: https://polarisproject.org/sites/default/files/Cantinas-SexTrafficking-EN.pdf. Accessed November 6, 2019.

Powell C, Asbill M, Louis E, et al: Identifying gaps in human trafficking mental health service provision. Journal of Human Trafficking 4(3):256–269, 2018

Rafferty Y: Mental health services as a vital component of psychosocial recovery for victims of child trafficking for commercial sexual exploitation. Am J Orthopsychiatry 88(3):249–260, 2017 30288452

Rajaram SS, Tidball S: Survivors' voices—complex needs of sex trafficking survivors in the Midwest. Behav Med 44(3):189–198, 2018 29095121

Rechtman R: Stories of trauma and idioms of distress: from cultural narratives to clinical assessment. Transcultural Psychiatry 37(3):403–198, 2000

Recknor FH, Gemeinhardt G, Selwyn BJ: Health-care provider challenges to the identification of human trafficking in health-care settings: a qualitative study. Journal of Human Trafficking 4(3):213–230, 2018

Reid JA: Entrapment and enmeshment schemes used by sex traffickers. Sex Abuse 28(6):491–511, 2016 25079777

Reid JA: Sex trafficking of girls with intellectual disabilities: An exploratory mixed methods study. Sex Abuse 30(2):107–131, 2018 26887695

Reid JA, Baglivio MT, Piquero AR, et al: Human trafficking of minors and childhood adversity in Florida. Am J Public Health 107(2):306–311, 2017 27997232

Ross C, Dimitrova S, Howard LM, et al: Human trafficking and health: a cross-sectional survey of NHS professionals' contact with victims of human trafficking. BMJ Open 5(8):e008682, 2015 26293659

Salami T, Gordon M, Coverdale J, et al: What therapies are favored in the treatment of the psychological sequelae of trauma in human trafficking victims? J Psychiatr Pract 24(2):87–96, 2018 29509178

Self-Brown S, Culbreth R, Wilson R, et al: Individual and parental risk factors for sexual exploitation among high-risk youth in Uganda. J Interpers Violence April 1, 2018 [Epub ahead of print] 29685056

Silverman JG, Decker MR, Gupta J, et al: Experiences of sex trafficking victims in Mumbai, India. Int J Gynecol Obstet 97(3):221–226, 2007a 17320087

Silverman JG, Decker MR, Gupta J, et al: HIV prevalence and predictors of infection in sex-trafficked Nepalese girls and women. JAMA 298(5):536–542, 2007b 17666674

Sprang G, Cole J: Familial sex trafficking of minors: trafficking conditions, clinical presentation, and system involvement. J Fam Violence 33(3):185–195, 2018

Steiner JJ, Kynn J, Stylianou AM, et al: Providing services to trafficking survivors: understanding practices across the globe. J Evid Inf Soc Work 15(2):150–168, 2018 29336727

Trafficking Victims Protection Act of 2000, Pub. L. No. 106-386 (22 U.S.C. § 7102). Available at: https://uscode.house.gov/view.xhtml?path=/prelim@title22/chapter78&edition=prelim. Accessed November 6, 2019.

UNICEF: Harrowing journeys: children and youth on the move across the Mediterranean Sea, at risk of trafficking and exploitation. September 2017. Available at: www.unicef.org/publications/files/Harrowing_Journeys_Children_and_youth_on_the_move_across_the_Mediterranean.pdf. Accessed November 6, 2019.

United Nations High Commissioner for Refugees: Children on the run: unaccompanied children leaving Central America and Mexico and the need for international protection. 2014. Available at: http://unhcr.org/en-us/about-us/background/56fc266f4/children-on-the-run-full-report.html. Accessed November 6, 2019.

United Nations Human Rights and Office of the High Commissioner for Human Rights: Convention on the rights of the child. 1990. Available at: http://ohchr.org/EN/ProfessionalInterest/Pages/CRC.aspx. Accessed November 6, 2019.

United Nations Human Rights and Office of the High Commissioner for Human Rights: Protocol to prevent, suppress and punish trafficking in persons, especially women and children, supplementing the United Nations Convention Against Transnational Organized Crime. November 15, 2000, Available at: https://ohchr.org/en/professionalinterest/pages/protocoltraffickinginpersons.aspx. Accessed July 7, 2017.

United Nations Office on Drugs and Crime: Global report on trafficking in persons. United Nations publications, Sales No. E.16.IV.6., 2016. Available at: http://unodc.org/documents/data-and-analysis/glotip/2016_Global_Report_on_Trafficking_in_Persons.pdf. Accessed November 6, 2019.

U.S. Department of State: Trafficking in persons report. June 2018. Available at: www.state.gov/wp-content/uploads/2019/01/282798.pdf. Accessed November 6, 2019.

van der Watt M, Kruger B: Exploring "juju" and human trafficking: towards a demystified perspective and response. South African Review of Sociology 48(2):70–86, 2017

Varma S, Gillespie S, McCracken C, et al: Characteristics of child commercial sexual exploitation and sex trafficking victims presenting for medical care in the United States. Child Abuse Negl 44:98–105, 2015 25896617

Viergever RF, West H, Borland R, et al: Health care providers and human trafficking: what do they know, what do they need to know? Findings from the Middle East, the Caribbean, and Central America. Front Public Health 3(6):6, 2015 25688343

Walls NE, Bell S: Correlates of engaging in survival sex among homeless youth and young adults. J Sex Res 48(5):423–436, 2011 20799134

West Coast Children's Clinic, National Center for Youth Law, Center for Trauma Recovery and Juvenile Justice: Psychotherapy for commercially sexually exploited children: a guide for community-based behavioral health practitioners and agencies. 2018. Available at: www.westcoastcc.org/wp-content/uploads/2018/10/MH_Treatment_Guide_CSEC.pdf. Accessed November 6, 2019.

Wolfe DS, Greerson JKP, Wasch S, et al: Human trafficking prevalence and child welfare risk factors among homeless youth: a multi-city study. The Field Center for Children's Policy, Practice, and Research, University of Pennsylvania, January 2018. Available at: https://fieldcenteratpenn.org/wp-content/uploads/2013/05/6230-R10-Field-Center-Full-Report-Web.pdf. Accessed November 6, 2019.

CHAPTER 12

Cultural Aspects in the Assessment and Management of Trafficked Persons

Ido Lurie, M.D., M.P.H.

Elana Cohn, M.D.

Ortal Slobodin, Ph.D.

I was a person who could no longer say "we" and who therefore said "I" merely out of habit, not now with the feeling of full possession of myself… I was no longer an I and did not live within a We. I had no passport, and no past, and no money, and no history. There was only a line of ancestors… and I had to take their ghosts along into exile… If I think back on the first days of exile in Antwerp, I still have the memory of a staggering on shaky ground. The mere fact that one could not decipher people's faces was frightening…Faces, gestures, clothes, houses, words (even if I halfway understood them) were sensory reality, but not interpretable signs. There was no order for me in this world…

I staggered through a world whose signs remained as inscrutable to me as Etruscan script. Unlike the tourist, however, for whom such things may be a piquant form of alienation, I was dependent on this world full of riddles. The man with the square skull, the police agent with the resentful voice…At times I felt more vulnerable before them than before the SS [Schutzstaffel] man at home; because of him I had at least known with

certainty that he was stupid and mean and that
he was after my life.

Jean Amery (1980)

A 19-year-old Eritrean asylum-seeker left her home country because
of the political situation: a military dictatorship took power and or-
dered much of the population into lifelong military service. Although
she had planned to emigrate to Europe, she was kidnapped and trafficked through the Sinai desert (Nakash et al. 2015). She was kept in
torture camps for 4 weeks, exposed to daily physical and sexual
abuse, including recurrent rapes, and was deprived of food and water. She was "sold" twice and was finally smuggled to the Egyptian-
Israeli border, only to be released after her relatives paid a high ran-
som fee for her freedom (about $30,000).

Once in Israel, after managing to make her way across the border
in 2012, she lived in a single-room apartment with 10 others in the
slums of Tel Aviv. Like many other asylum-seekers in Israel, she had
only a temporary visa, which did not allow her any welfare or health
rights (for further details, see Lurie and Nakash 2015). She could
hardly work because of her physical and mental condition, only managing to work as a waitress part-time in an Eritrean bar, where male
clients continually physically harassed her.

After almost 2 years in Israel, she arrived at the *Gesher* (Bridge
in English) clinic, an established free governmental psychiatric clinic
for asylum-seekers and trafficked persons (Lurie 2017). On her first
intake evaluation, she reported low energy, insomnia, despair, and
mainly unexplained somatic symptoms (stomach, back, head, and
limb aches). As the therapist knew about the torture camps in Sinai,
the patient was delicately asked about such experiences. However,
she was ashamed and reluctant to disclose any such experiences because she was afraid that her relatives would find out. In the Eritrean patriarchal community, it is difficult to discuss the issues of
rape and sexual assault, for both men and women. Rape is considered a taboo topic of conversation by Eritreans, and rape victims are
usually accused of responsibility for their misfortune.

Initially, the patient was diagnosed with depression with somatic
features, with suspicion of PTSD. Although she refused any psychiatric medication, she did agree to psychosocial intervention with a
social worker. At the beginning, the appointments were directive and
supportive. She was taught cognitive and relaxation techniques, and
her weekly schedule was reviewed. With behavioral activation interventions, she was encouraged and able to function at home and at
work, and her somatic symptoms decreased. She gradually became
attached to her therapist and began to trust her. The patient disclosed feelings of loneliness, detachment, and alienation. She needed
someone to talk to and share her life with.

After about 6 months of weekly appointments, she finally revealed the story of her kidnaping in Sinai. The accepting response of

her social worker, and, moreover, of the Eritrean interpreter, led to a substantial improvement in her condition. Although it was difficult to convince her that reporting her kidnapping and trafficking experience would benefit her—human trafficking survivors in Israel are granted rehabilitation, economic, and housing services—she ultimately agreed.[1]

In this chapter we outline the relevance and importance of cultural aspects for mental health experts who work with trafficked persons. We then describe various cultural complexities in the diagnosis and treatment of trafficked persons, with potential pitfalls and special considerations. We close the chapter with a discussion of interventions that require cultural sensitivity, including psychotherapy, pharmacotherapy, and community interventions.

IMPORTANCE OF CONSIDERING CULTURE IN WORKING WITH TRAFFICKED PERSONS

In a time of ever-growing global migration and blending of communities, cultural competency in medicine—and specifically in mental health—is of the utmost necessity. In 2017, there were known to be 258 million immigrants, equaling over 3% of the world's population (United Nations 2017). Of them, about 72% were considered international migrants, and women made up 48% of all international migrants worldwide. Human trafficking often involves migration to a different country, as noted: "trafficking in persons" is defined as "the recruitment, transportation, transfer, harbouring or receipt of persons, by means of the threat or use of force or other forms of coercion …" (United Nations Office on Drugs and Crime 2000).

However, the delineation between these vulnerable groups of migrants (e.g., human trafficking survivors, refugees, asylum-seekers, work migrants) is gradually converging, and these vulnerable groups are referred to by the term *forced migrants* (Burnett and Ndovi 2018; International Organization for Migration 2019).

The migration process involves three stages: 1) premigration, 2) migration, and 3) postmigration. Each stage involves significant risks for emotional distress and the development of diagnosable psychiatric disorders (Bhugra et al. 2011). Therefore, immigration by itself is con-

---

[1]The authors would like to thank Shlomit Ben Shmuel, M.S.W., for her contribution of this clinical vignette.

sidered a risk factor for mental health problems (Kirmayer et al. 2011). Moreover, whether it be in their country of origin, during the migration process, or in their new host country/society, forced migrants are likely to be subjected to a multitude of traumatic physical, sexual, psychological, and spiritual experiences (Greenbaum 2017). Trafficked persons may undergo prolonged situations of abuse, exposure to violence, dependence on a dominant person(s), kidnapping, smuggling, and/or imprisonment. The impact of these traumatic experiences is typically exacerbated by the challenges of adjustment to a new culture and fear of losing their identity (Sue and Sue 2016). Other documented independent risk factors for mental disorders include childhood sexual abuse, long duration of trafficking, and an increased number of unmet needs posttrafficking (Abas et al. 2013).

As a result of these traumatic experiences, trafficked persons are at increased risk for emotional distress and psychiatric symptoms and disorders, including depression, anxiety, PTSD, psychosomatic disorders, psychosis, eating disorders, and substance abuse (as self-medication), as well as self-injurious behavior and suicidality (Anna-Clara et al. 2016; Edinburgh et al. 2015; Goldberg et al. 2017; Hollander et al. 2016; Lindert et al. 2009; Tsutsumi et al. 2008; Zimmerman et al. 2008). Psychological manifestations of the prolonged trafficking process may include identification with the aggressor, denial, and learned helplessness. For some trafficked persons, the trauma of trafficking and abuse was inflicted by someone they trusted. This may result in pervasive mistrust of others and their motives. In her seminal book *Trauma and Recovery*, Judith Herman (1992, p. 116) concluded the following: "While it is clear that ordinary, healthy people may become entrapped in prolonged abusive situations, it is equally clear that after their escape they are no longer ordinary or healthy. Chronic abuse causes serious psychological harm."

CULTURAL CONSIDERATIONS AND COMPLEXITIES IN DIAGNOSIS AND TREATMENT OF TRAFFICKED PERSONS

The unique culture of origin of each micropopulation shapes and influences the communication of traumas and their psychological and psychiatric sequalae, as well as the behavior and expectations of those seeking treatment (Qureshi et al. 2015). Culture also shapes the models clinicians use to interpret the patient's history in terms of psychiatric diagnoses (Kleinman 1987). Because the psychiatric diagnosis process is somewhat subjective, phenomenology based, and deeply immersed in cultural context (Lewis-Fernández and Aggarwal 2013), when the patient and the therapist do not share the same cultural and linguistic background, the whole process of diagnosis and the tailoring of the psychiatric and psychosocial treatment plan is prone to pitfalls. This was described by Kleinman (1987) as *category fallacy*—that is, applying a diagnostic category that is valid in one cultural context (e.g., Western psychiatric nosology) to a culture in which the category has no local relevance or diagnostic validity.

As noted earlier in this chapter (see section "Importance of Considering Culture in Working With Trafficked Persons"), mental manifestations—as well as the patient's resilience and other individual factors—may present in various and diverse manners according to one's culture. When working in a cross-cultural environment, there are several important issues to consider for the therapeutic process, communication, diagnostic evaluation, and, later, the tailoring of treatment planning.

Diagnostic Mismatch

During the clinical interview, the clinician is looking for a diagnostic syndrome or disorder (which is a cultural construct), while the patient's idioms of distress are molded by his or her culture of origin. The expression of distress may be conceptualized and labeled as pathological by the clinician but may not be truly related to any psychopathology.

Communication and Language Barriers

Language is at the heart of mental health care (Swartz et al. 2014). Limited language proficiency and language barriers are problematic, specifically to mental health care. Psychiatric or psychological evaluation hinges on obtaining a thorough history (anamnesis), because most of the key symptoms and signs are not directly observable and they can be elicited only via communication and self-report (Bauer and Alegría 2010). Physical examination and further laboratory and imaging testing are of limited utility, typically helpful only to rule out organic diagnoses or contributors. Therefore, most mental health diagnoses and treatments rely on direct communication rather than objective tests or biological treatments (Sentell et al. 2007). The language barrier may lead to incorrect details in history taking, increased risk of misdiagnosis, difficulty in conveying delicate emotions in a tongue that is not the first language of the patient, underestimation of adaptation abilities and cognitive executive functions, and limited ability to establish emotional communication and rapport. This may endanger the trust development process and the whole therapeutic course. In a review of challenges faced by mental health providers in the United States treating elderly immigrants, language barriers were described as the major source of difficulty in providing services (Weisman et al. 2005).

Diagnostic Considerations

In psychiatry, the mental status examination (MSE) constitutes a central component of diagnosis. The MSE is based on observation and interpretation of the patient's behavior and mental activity—both spontaneous and as elicited by questions. However, when the clinician and the patient are from different cultures, the interpretation of every aspect of the MSE requires caution, as it may be distorted and culturally biased. Thus, the psychiatric evaluation should consider the patient's own culturally normative framework as a referent. All testing instruments and evaluation tools should be normed with the patient's cultural group and externally validated to that group to ensure reliability and validity of the assessment.

Traumatic History

In any therapeutic setting, but especially in working with trafficked persons, there is often a lack of spontaneous talk about experiences of trauma (Nordstrom 2004). This may be secondary to a strongly held cultural value of privacy or a result of a cultural difference in which flashbacks or nightmares are not thought to be related to trauma (Chung et al. 2007; Schouler-Ocak 2015). A lack of spontaneous discussion is further worsened by the fact that providers do not frequently ask the appropriate questions (Al-Saffar et al. 2004; Shannon et al. 2012). In response, patients often may not bring up the trauma in deference to the primary care doctor's authority, creating a destructive cycle. The most difficult/complicated barrier to overcome is a generalized lack of trust in the health care system because of the traumatic effect of previous providers using health care as a form of control or torture in their home country (Asner-Self et al. 2005).

Mental Health Literacy

Persons from different cultures and origins may have different concepts and models regarding mental health diagnoses and health services. Health illiteracy and atypical idioms of distress (Kirmayer and Young 1998) may prevent access to services or limit benefit from treatment.

Culture and cultural gaps between patient and therapist may be even more important in trafficked persons for several reasons. First, cultural differences in symptom manifestation result in major difficulties in understanding symptoms and building therapeutic alignment and alliance (Bhatia and Wallace 2007; van Loon et al. 2011). Cultural competence is particularly crucial when discrimination and racism are the foci of treatment because the role of the professional's race, sexual orientation, ethnicity, and gender are often magnified in treatment (Dunbar 2001). Second, many trafficked persons—and among them specific populations such as refugees—are affiliated with collective cultures, and their core traumas likely involve attacks on collective identity. In situations involving ethnic persecution or political violence, people may become victims of trauma simply by belonging to a certain cultural group (Bryant-Davis and Tummala-Narra 2017), so the trauma itself may be perceived through the community's lens (Kira et al. 2010). Third, the act of human trafficking is heavily influenced by cultural norms and values, such as gender or ethnic stereotypes. For example, gender stereotypes that present men as powerful and active and women as passive and limited to the domestic sphere contribute to the common misconception that "men migrate, but women are trafficked." These cultural norms fail to recognize that men too are trafficked and that women not only are trafficked but also migrate (R. Sengupta, S. Huq, "Trafficking of Persons and Gender Inequality in South Asia," unpublished paper, 2001). Finally, human trafficking has negative effects not only on mental health and interpersonal relations but also on communal and cultural systems (e.g., loss of social solidarity, increase of ethnic hate, increase of distrust). Therefore, the reestablishment of cultural identity may be considered as a key resource area in improving the psychosocial well-being of trafficked victims.

Up-to-date studies with diverse samples of trafficked persons have repeatedly revealed poor cultural sensitivity in the treatment setting. For example, in qualitative work by Aron et al. (2006), trafficked persons described wanting other services, outside of one-to-one therapy, to address their emotional needs (e.g., acupuncture). In addition, victims described their experiences of one-to-one therapy as often shameful and blaming, and they found that Western style talk therapy did not always resonate with their cultural backgrounds (Kung 2014; Macy and Johns 2011). This lack of cultural sensitivity, coupled with the worldwide increasing prevalence of human trafficking victims, emphasizes the ethical and scientific imperative of developing a culturally sensitive approach in all areas of mental health, including diagnostic tools, monitoring, evaluation, and interagency cooperation (Hinton and Jalal 2014; Hobfoll and de Jong 2014).

A possible framework for employing the diagnostic process of mental disorders in trafficked persons should include three parallel (yet not completely separate) arms (as detailed in Figure 12–1): 1) Western-oriented diagnosis, according to DSM-5 (American Psychiatric Association 2013) or ICD-10 (World Health Organization 1993); 2) a cultural diagnostic approach (e.g., the Cultural Formulation Interview, DSM-5; Lewis-Fernández et al. 2014), which is based on understanding symptoms in the context of the patient's culture of origin and his or her narrative; and 3) persistent yet considerate attempts to screen for undisclosed past and current traumatic exposure(s), losses, and posttraumatic symptoms, related to all stages of the trafficking process and migration.

MANAGEMENT OF CULTURAL COMPLEXITY

General Considerations

Working with trafficked persons should follow general considerations according to the biopsychosocial model (Figure 12–1). However, there are various pathways through which culture can be incorporated into mental health services for trafficked persons. Certain cultural and language barriers could be overcome by working with interpreters and cultural mediators/brokers. A professional interpreter could facilitate the disclosure of victims' experiences, help build trust, and support the trafficked person in navigating health services (Lederer and Wetzel 2014). Working with interpreters involves some potential (or perceived) difficulties, including confidentiality, stigma, and embarrassment (Patel et al. 2010). For instance, several authors highlighted the importance of providing female-only services for female trafficked persons because of their reluctance to speak about sexual health problems with a male doctor, mental health professional, or an interpreter (Chisolm-Straker et al. 2012; Zimmerman et al. 2003). However, female-only services may not be available for every clinical setting.

When therapists are working with interpreters, there are several important issues. First, laypersons from the same trafficked per-

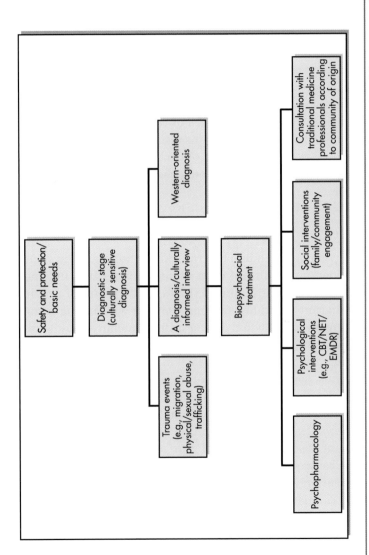

FIGURE 12–1. A culturally sensitive treatment approach for the mental health needs of human trafficking victims.

CBT=cognitive-behavioral therapy; EMDR=eye movement desensitization and reprocessing; NET=narrative exposure therapy.

sons' community who work as interpreters in mental health settings must have some training. This training should include an under-standing of mental health concepts and issues (at least in Western terminology) as well as of medical ethics, including an understand-ing of medical confidentiality, patient autonomy, and informed con-sent. Second, it is advisable that interpreters in mental health have ongoing supervision, either by an individual and/or group. This may reduce burnout and secondary traumatization and ensure continu-ous improvement of services. Third, once the therapeutic triad is set, it is highly important to work with the same interpreter over time as much as possible.

Because of the traumatic nature of the trafficking process and cultural complexities and barriers (as discussed), the therapist must be willing to allow a longer period of time for a full detailed history to be disclosed by building trust and a therapeutic alliance.

Individual Treatment

Psychosocial Interventions

The intersection between human trafficking and migration requires not only strong multicultural counseling competencies, in general, but also a deep understanding of the distinct nature of providing care to immigrant individuals. When working with immigrants, es-pecially refugees and asylum-seekers, the clinician should address the adverse premigration and postmigration experiences of the pa-tient, including persecution, war, lack of social support, accultura-tion difficulties, poverty, discrimination, and changes in identity and concept of self (Bhugra and Becker 2005; Laban et al. 2004).

Researchers and clinicians have long debated whether trauma-focused interventions, such as cognitive-behavioral therapy (CBT) or eye movement desensitization and reprocessing (EMDR), are appli-cable to the refugee population or whether a phased model starting with stabilization is preferable. Some clinicians (e.g., Başoğlu 2006) argue that traumatized refugees should be treated according to the standardized protocols of CBT and EMDR, but others (Laban et al. 2009; National Institute for Health and Clinical Excellence 2005) contend that treatment should start with a restoration of coping skills and dealing with daily stressors. Culturally adapted trauma-focused interventions such as CBT and narrative exposure therapy (NET) have been found to be effective in reducing symptoms of PTSD in refugee patients (for review, see Slobodin and de Jong 2015b). An-other possible approach (for both individual and group therapy) is

EMDR therapy (Altun et al. 2017). Nevertheless, the acceptability of these treatments among trafficked people is unknown, as is the generalizability of therapies effective for other traumatized groups such as victims of domestic violence (Hemmings et al. 2016). Often, traumatized individuals tend to feel ambivalent about engaging in psychosocial intervention, mainly because of a fear of repatriation (Vincent et al. 2013). Using the principles of motivational interviewing may enhance patients' motivation for change and assist in establishing trust. Motivational interviewing builds on Carl Rogers' optimistic and humanistic theories about people's capabilities for exercising free choice and changing through a process of self-actualization (Rogers 1959). This counseling style assumes that ambivalence about change is normal and constitutes an important motivational obstacle in recovery. The therapeutic relationship is considered a democratic, collaborative partnership to which each part brings important expertise. The therapist should empathically uncover any discrepancy between clients' goals or values and their current behavior, adjust to client resistance rather than opposing it directly, and support self-efficacy and optimism in the client (Miller and Rollnick 1991).

Psychopharmacotherapy

When clinicians are considering medication for trafficked persons, it is necessary to remember that different cultures may have different attitudes and beliefs toward psychopharmacotherapy, its therapeutic and placebo effects, all of which influence individuals' acceptance of and adherence to medication (De Las Cuevas et al. 2018; Schomerus et al. 2014). Different attitudes include stigma, skepticism, pharmacophobia, and pharmacophilia. Initial assessment and understanding of patients' attitudes toward psychiatric drug treatment by clinicians may improve patients' confidence and overall adherence to prescribed treatment and may enhance the therapeutic alliance and allow for better tailoring of medical treatment and optimization of treatment outcomes.

Group and Community Interventions

Human trafficking involves a massive disruption of social networks due to loss, displacement, and distrust (Silove et al. 2017). Therefore, community-based interventions may provide an optimal strategy to reestablish meaning and agency (Inter-Agency Standing Committee 2006). The World Health Organization (2016) recommends an increase in the use of mental health interventions in communities with limited resources by implementing "task shifting" in which interventions are provided by lay counselors in primary or community settings.

Group interventions may provide an opportunity to discuss how other people have dealt with adversity. Cultural themes of resilience may be incorporated in folk stories, art, literature, music, or culturally proscribed traditions to solve problems (Dunbar 2001). Given the importance of the family in the aftermath of human trafficking and the theoretical ease of including the social and cultural context in systemic approaches to therapy (Mendenhall and Berge 2010; Slobodin and de Jong 2015a), family interventions or multifamily groups should also be considered (Birman et al. 2008). Nevertheless, group interventions should be used with caution in the context of human trafficking, as they may have negative results. For example, individuals who have been trafficked may have been encouraged by their traffickers to compete with others who were trafficked or, in some cases, participate in their abuse. In addition, significant cultural and social divides, as well as fear of being found by their trafficking network, may prevent victims of trafficking from trusting other victims (Shigekane 2007).

Developing Culturally Informed Interventions

Studies with ethnic minorities, refugees, and people in low-income countries suggest that culturally informed psychosocial interventions require a global and local understanding of mental health issues (e.g., cultural idioms of distress, protective and resilience factors, help-seeking behaviors) as well as knowledge about the expectations and preferences of the affected population (Hinton et al. 2004, 2008; Tol et al. 2014). Jordans et al. (2011) presented a research strategy aimed at facilitating informed decision-making for selecting interventions within low- and middle-income countries. The model assumes that because evidence-based treatment from high-income settings cannot be simply transferred to low- and middle-income countries (Patel 2009), a preliminary cultural adaptation stage is needed. This adaptation stage comprises four phases: a qualitative phase to assess needs and determine tentative intervention objectives; an exploratory phase in which a global panel of experts identifies intervention modalities for low-resource settings; a phase including both a systematic literature review and a distillation of practice elements from evidence-based treatments; and a phase consisting of stakeholder meetings to examine social-cultural feasibility and acceptability of the developed intervention (Jordans et al. 2011). Drawing on this model, Slobodin et al. (2018) used focus group discussions in order to develop a culturally sensitive psychosocial intervention for asylum-seekers in the Netherlands. Analysis of qualitative data collected during focus group discussions with Syrian asylum-seekers revealed that mental health problems were more frequently associated with postmigration stressors (e.g., identity loss, uncertainty, helplessness) than with past traumatic experiences. In addition, individuals and communities appeared to be limited in their ability to provide support for those suffering from psychosocial distress because of the heavy stigma related to mental health issues and the burden of multiple stressors.

CONCLUSION

Trafficked persons are at increased risk for emotional distress and psychiatric diagnoses, which may have different manifestations according to the individual's culture. Therefore, culturally informed diagnostic processes and culturally sensitive interventions on individual, group, and community levels are recommended to optimize the recovery process.

Pearls and Pointers

- Clinicians should be aware of and sensitive to cultural differences and diversities throughout all levels of service (administrative, clinical evaluation, and psychosocial interventions).

- Information about the potential advantages of mental health intervention should be presented and explained in comprehensible terms. Clinicians should avoid imposing preconceived notions, judgments, and labels on behaviors with which they may not be familiar.

- Clinicians should establish empathy and rapport; be humble and respectful. If clinicians do not know something, they should ask in a sensitive manner. It may be useful to ask for the patient's explanation for their distress or illness.

- Safety, protection, and practical considerations should be prioritized (e.g., food, shelter, clothing). Consider helping with legal protection and a temporary status visa.

- Sufficient time should be allowed for patients to recover. Clinicians should maintain patience for dealing with prolonged trust issues and should approach patients with a trauma-informed care model.

- Clinicians should work with cultural consultants/brokers whose backgrounds reflect the trafficked person's culture and community.

- Clinicians should ask about all stages of trafficking: pretrafficking, the trafficking process, and posttrafficking conditions.

- Clinicians should acquire information regarding the culture and the background of the patients by focusing on the narrative. The patient's story should be used as a tool to create a shared world of assumptions and values to establish a fuller context on all three stages of trafficking.

REFERENCES

Abas M, Ostrovschi NV, Prince M, et al: Risk factors for mental disorders in women survivors of human trafficking: a historical cohort study. BMC Psychiatry 13(1):204, 2013 23914952

Al-Saffar S, Borgå P, Wicks S, Hällström T: The influence of the patients' ethnicity, sociodemographic conditions and strain on psychiatric diagnoses given at an outpatient clinic. Nord J Psychiatry 58(6):421–427, 2004 16195085

Altun S, Abas M, Zimmerman C, et al: Mental health and human trafficking: responding to survivors' needs. BJPsych Int 14(1):21–23, 2017 29093930

American Psychiatric Association: Diagnostic and Statistical Manual of Mental Disorders, 5th Edition. Arlington, VA, American Psychiatric Association, 2013

Amery J: At the Mind's Limits: Contemplations by a Survivor on Auschwitz and Its Realities. Bloomington, IN, Indiana University Press, 1980, pp 44–47

Anna-Clara H, Dal Henrik LG, Cecilia M, et al: Refugee migration and risk of schizophrenia and other non-affective psychoses: cohort study of 1.3 million people in Sweden. BMJ 352:i1030, 2016 23914952

Aron LY, Zweig JM, Newmark LS: Comprehensive Services for Survivors of Human Trafficking: Findings From Clients in Three Communities. Washington, DC, Urban Institute, 2006

Aronowitz AA: The social etiology of human trafficking: how poverty and cultural practices facilitate trafficking. Paper presented at the Pontifical Academy of Social Sciences Human Trafficking: Issues Beyond Criminalization, April 2015 Casina Pio IV, Vatican City, 2015

Asner-Self KK, Marotta SA: Developmental indices among Central American immigrants exposed to war-related trauma: clinical implications for counselors. Journal of Counseling and Development 83:162–171, 2005

Başoğlu M: Rehabilitation of traumatised refugees and survivors of torture. BMJ 333(7581):1230–1231, 2006 17170393

Bauer AM, Alegría M: Impact of patient language proficiency and interpreter service use on the quality of psychiatric care: a systematic review. Psychiatr Serv 61(8):765–773, 2010 20675834

Bhatia R, Wallace P: Experiences of refugees and asylum seekers in general practice: a qualitative study. BMC Fam Pract 8:48–56, 2007 17711587

Bhugra D, Becker MA: Migration, cultural bereavement and cultural identity. World Psychiatry 4(1):18–24, 2005 16633496

Bhugra D, Gupta S, Bhui K, et al: WPA guidance on mental health and mental health care in migrants. World Psychiatry 10(1):2–10, 2011 21379345

Birman D, Beehler S, Harris EM, et al: International family, adult, and child enhancement services (FACES): a community-based comprehensive services model for refugee children in resettlement. Am J Orthopsychiatry 78(1):121–132, 2008 18444734

Bryant-Davis T, Tummala-Narra U: Cultural oppression and human trafficking: exploring the role of racism and ethnic bias. Women and Therapy 40:(1–2):152–169, 2017

Burnett A, Ndovi T: The health of forced migrants. BMJ 328:(7446):1013–1014, 2018 151055330

Chisolm-Straker M, Richardson LD, Cossio T: Combating slavery in the 21st century: the role of emergency medicine. J Health Care Poor Underserved 23(3):980–987, 2012 24212151

Chung RC-Y, Bemak F, Talleyrand RM: Mentoring within the field of counseling: a preliminary study of multicultural perspectives. International Journal for the Advancement of Counselling 29(1):21–32, 2007

De Las Cuevas C, Motuca M, Baptista T, et al: Skepticism and pharmacophobia toward medication may negatively impact adherence to psychiatric medications: a comparison among outpatient samples recruited in Spain, Argentina, and Venezuela. Patient Prefer Adherence 12:301–310, 2018 29503532

Dunbar E: Counseling practices to ameliorate the effects of discrimination and hate events: toward a systematic approach to assessment and intervention. The Counseling Psychologist 29:279–307, 2001

Edinburgh L, Pape-Blabolil J, Harpin SB, et al: Assessing exploitation experiences of girls and boys seen at a child advocacy center. Child Abuse Neglect 46:47–59, 2015 25982287

Goldberg AP, Moore JL, Houck C, et al: Domestic minor sex trafficking patients: a retrospective analysis of medical presentation. J Pediatr Adolesc Gynecol 30(1):109–115, 2017 27575407

Greenbaum VJ: Child sex trafficking in the United States: challenges for the healthcare provider. PLoS Med 14(11):e1002439, 2017 29166405

Hemmings S, Jakobowitz S, Abas M, et al: Responding to the health needs of survivors of human trafficking: a systematic review. BMC Health Serv Res 16(16):320, 2016 27473258

Herman JL: Trauma and Recovery: The Aftermath of Violence—From Domestic Abuse to Political Terror. New York, Basic Books, 1992

Hinton DE, Jalal B: Guidelines for the implementation of culturally sensitive cognitive behavioural therapy among refugees and in global contexts., Intervention: International Journal of Mental Health. Psychosocial Work and Counselling in Areas of Armed Conflict 12:78–79, 2014

Hinton DE, Pham T, Tran M, et al: CBT for Vietnamese refugees with treatment-resistant PTSD and panic attacks: a pilot study. J Trauma Stress 17(5):429–433, 2004 15633922

Hinton DE, Hofmann SG, Pitman RK, et al: The panic attack-posttraumatic stress disorder model: applicability to orthostatic panic among Cambodian refugees. Cogn Behav Ther 37(2):101–116, 2008 18470741

Hobfoll SE, de Jong TVMJ: The course and limitations of natural recovery from trauma: the centrality of threats to attachment and safety and their reinstatement, in Facilitating Resilience and Recovery Following Traumatic Events. Edited by Zoellner LA, Feeny NC. New York, Guilford, 2014, pp 69–89

Hollander AC, Dal H, Lewis G, et al: Refugee migration and risk of schizophrenia and other non-affective psychoses: cohort study of 1.3 million people in Sweden. BMJ 352:i1030, Mar 15, 2016 26979256 [Erratum in BMJ 353:i2865, May 27, 2016]

Inter-Agency Standing Committee: IASC guidelines for gender-based violence: interventions in humanitarian settings. 2006. Available at: www.paho.org/hq/dmdocuments/2010/GBV_humanitarian_settings.pdf. Accessed November 7, 2019.

International Organization for Migration: Displacement, forced migration. Glossary on Migration, 2019. Available at: https://migrationdataportal.org/themes/forced-migration-or-displacement#data-sources. Accessed November 7, 2019.

Jordans MJD, Tol WA, Komproe IH: Mental health interventions for children in adversity: pilot-testing a research strategy for treatment selection in low-income settings. Soc Sci Med 73(3):456–466, 2011 21742426

Kira IA, Ahmed A, Mahmoud V, et al: Group therapy model for refugee and torture survivors. Torture 20(2):108–113, 2010 20952827

Kirmayer LJ, Young A: Culture and somatization: clinical, epidemiological, and ethnographic perspectives. Psychosom Med 60(4):420–430, 1998 9710287

Kirmayer LJ, Narasiah L, Munoz M, et al; Canadian Collaboration for Immigrant and Refugee Health (CCIRH): Common mental health problems in immigrants and refugees: general approach in primary care. CMAJ 183(12):E959–E967, 2011 20603342

Kleinman A: Anthropology and psychiatry. The role of culture in cross-cultural research on illness. Br J Psychiatry 151(4):447–454, 1987 3447661

Kung J: Sex trafficking: an exploration of clinician perspectives of the type and efficacy of treatment interventions. Smith College—Theses, Dissertations, and Projects, 2014. Available at: https://pdfs.semanticscholar.org/c160/1cd63609e675d3165f0858c96ff4fd4aa87f.pdf. Accessed November 6, 2019.

Laban CJ, Gernaat HB, Komproe IH, et al: Impact of a long asylum procedure on the prevalence of psychiatric disorders in Iraqi asylum seekers in The Netherlands. J Nerv Ment Dis 192(12):843–851, 2004 15583506

Laban CJ, Hurulean E, Attia A: Treatment of asylum seekers: resilience-oriented therapy and strategies (ROTS): implications of study results into clinical practice, in Handboek Culturele Psychiatrie en Psychotherapie. Edited by de Joop J, Colijn S. Utrecht, The Netherlands, De Tijdstroom, 2009, pp 127–146

Lederer LJ, Wetzel CA: The health consequences of sex trafficking and their implications for identifying victims in healthcare facilities. Annals of Health Law 23(1):61–87, 2014

Lewis-Fernández R, Aggarwal NK: Culture and psychiatric diagnosis. Adv Psychosom Med 33:15–30, 2013 23816860

Lewis-Fernández R, Aggarwal NK, Bäärnhielm S, et al: Culture and psychiatric evaluation: operationalizing cultural formulation for DSM-5. Psychiatry 77(2):130–154, 2014 24865197

Lindert J, von Ehrenstein OS, Priebe S, et al: Depression and anxiety in labor migrants and refugees: a systematic review and meta-analysis. Soc Sci Med 69(2):246–257, 2009 19539414

Lurie I: The mental health of asylum seekers and victims of human trafficking: the experience of Gesher (Bridge) clinic, Israel 2014–2017, in symposium: psychiatric experience in the treatment of genocide and torture surviving refugees (S-227). Presented at the World Congress of Psychiatry, World Psychiatric Association XVII, Berlin, October 8–12, 2017

Lurie I, Nakash O: Exposure to trauma and forced migration: mental health and acculturation patterns among asylum seekers in Israel, in Trauma and Migration: Cultural Factors in the Diagnosis and Treatment of Traumatised Immigrants. Edited by Schouler-Ocak M. New York, Springer, 2015, pp 139–156

Macy RJ, Johns N: Aftercare services for international sex trafficking survivors: informing U.S. service and program development in an emerging practice area. Trauma Violence Abuse 12(2):87–98, 2011 21196435

Mendenhall TJ, Berge JM: Family therapists in trauma-response teams: bringing systems thinking into interdisciplinary fieldwork. Journal of Family Therapy 32:43–57, 2010

Miller WR, Rollnick S: Motivational Interviewing: Preparing People to Change Addictive Behavior. New York, Guilford, 1991

Nakash O, Langer B, Nagar M, et al: Exposure to traumatic experiences among asylum seekers from Eritrea and Sudan during migration to Israel. J Immigr Minor Health 17(4):1280–1286, 2015 24752982

National Institute for Health and Clinical Excellence: Post-traumatic Stress Disorder (PTSD): The Management of PTSD in Adults and Children in Primary and Secondary Care. London, National Institute for Health and Clinical Excellence, 2005

Nordstrom C: Shadows of War: Violence, Power, and International Profiteering in the Twenty-First Century. Berkeley, University of California Press, 2004

Patel RB, Ahn R, Burke TF: Human trafficking in the emergency department. West J Emerg Med 11(5):402–404, 2010 21293753

Patel V: The future of psychiatry in low- and middle-income countries. Psychol Med 39(11):1759–1762, 2009 20162837

Qureshi A, Bague IF, Ghali K, et al: Cultural competence in trauma, in Trauma and Migration: Cultural Factors in the Diagnosis and Treatment of Traumatized Immigrants. Cham, Switzerland, Springer International Publishing, 2015, pp 159–172

Rogers CR: A theory of therapy, personality, and interpersonal relationships: as developed in the client-centered framework, in Psychology: A Study of a Science, Vol 3: Formulations of the Person and the Social Context. Edited by Koch S. New York, McGraw-Hill, 1959, pp 184–256

Schomerus G, Matschinger H, Baumeister SE, et al: Public attitudes towards psychiatric medication: a comparison between United States and Germany. World Psychiatry 13(3):320–321, 2014 25273308

Schouler-Ocak M (ed): Trauma and Migration: Cultural Factors in the Diagnosis and Treatment of Traumatised Immigrants. New York, Springer, 2015

Sentell T, Shumway M, Snowden L: Access to mental health treatment by English language proficiency and race/ethnicity. J Gen Intern Med 22(2)(Suppl 2):289–293, 2007 17957413

Shannon P, O'Dougherty M, Mehta E: Refugees' perspectives on barriers to communication about trauma histories in primary care. Ment Health Fam Med 9(1):47–55, 2012 23277798

Shigekane R: Rehabilitation and community integration of trafficking survivors in the United States. . Human Rights Quarterly 29:112–136, 2007

Silove D, Ventevogel P, Rees S: The contemporary refugee crisis: an overview of mental health challenges. World Psychiatry 16(2):130–139, 2017 28498581

Slobodin O, de Jong JTVM: Family interventions in traumatized immigrants and refugees: a systematic review. Transcult Psychiatry 52(6):723–742, 2015a 26047828

Slobodin O, de Jong JTVM: Mental health interventions for traumatized asylum seekers and refugees: what do we know about their efficacy? Int J Soc Psychiatry 61(1):17–26, 2015b 24869847

Slobodin O, Ghane S, de Jong JTVM: Developing a culturally sensitive mental health intervention for asylum seekers in the Netherlands. Intervention 16(2):86–94, 2018

Sue DW, Sue D: Counseling the Culturally Diverse: Theory and Practice, 7th Edition, Hoboken, NJ, Wiley, 2016, pp 591–612

Swartz L, Kilian S, Twesigye J, et al: Language, culture, and task shifting—an emerging challenge for global mental health. Glob Health Action 7:23433, 2014 24581319

Tol WA, Komproe IH, Jordans MJ, et al: School-based mental health intervention for children in war affected Burundi: a cluster randomized trial. BMC Medicine 12:56, 2014 24690470

Tsutsumi A, Izutsu T, Poudyal AK, et al: Mental health of female survivors of human trafficking in Nepal. Soc Sci Med 66(8):1841–1847, 2008 18276050

United Nations: International migration report. Department of Economic and Social Affairs, Population Division, 2017. Available at: www.un.org/en/development/desa/population/migration/publications/migrationreport/docs/MigrationReport2017.pdf. Accessed November 7, 2019.

United Nations Office on Drugs and Crime: Protocol to Prevent, Suppress and Punish Trafficking in Persons, Especially Women and Children, supplementing the United Nations Convention against Transnational Organized Crime. Annex 2, Article 3. Vienna, United Nations, 2000. Available at: https://unodc.org/documents/treaties/UNTOC/Publications/TOC%20Convention/TOCebook-e.pdf. Accessed February 24, 2020.

Vincent F, Jenkins H, Larkin M, et al: Asylum seekers' experiences of trauma-focused cognitive behaviour therapy for posttraumatic stress disorder: a qualitative study. Behav Cogn Psychother 41(5):579–593, 2013 22794141

Weine S, Kulauzovic Y, Klebuc A, et al: Evaluating a multiple-family group access intervention for refugees with PTSD. J Marital Fam Ther 34(2):149–164, 2008 18412823

Weisman A, Feldman G, Gruman C, et al: Improving mental health services for Latino and Asian immigrant elders. Professional Psychology: Research and Practice 36:642–648, 2005

World Health Organization: The ICD-10 Classification of Mental and Behavioural Disorders: Diagnostic Criteria for Research. Geneva, World Health Organization, 1993

World Health Organization: Problem Management Plus (PM+). Individual Psychological Help for Adults Impaired by Distress in Communities Exposed to Adversity. (Generic Field-Trial Version 1.0). Geneva, World Health Organization, 2016

van Loon A, van Schaik DJF, Dekker JJ, et al: Effectiveness of an intercultural module added to the treatment guidelines for Moroccan and Turkish patients with depressive and anxiety disorders. BMC Psychiatry 11:13–19, 2011 21247455

Zimmerman C, Yun K, Shvab I, et al: The health risks and consequences of trafficking in women and adolescents: findings from a European study. London School of Hygiene and Tropical Medicine, 2003. Available at: https://researchonline.lshtm.ac.uk/id/eprint/10786. Accessed November 7, 2019.

Zimmerman C, Hossain M, Yun K, et al: The health of trafficked women: a survey of women entering posttrafficking services in Europe. Am J Public Health 98(1):55–59, 2008 18048781

CHAPTER 13

The Clinician as Advocate

CONFIDENTIALITY AND REPORTING
REQUIREMENTS

Shea M. Rhodes, J.D.

Stephanie Mersch

> We have been called to heal wounds, to unite
> what has fallen away, and to bring home those
> who have lost their way.
>
> —*St. Francis of Assisi*

Navigating complex patient confidentiality and child abuse reporting requirements to best serve trafficked persons can seem like a
daunting task filled with legal jargon. However, there are many resources available to clinicians to assist you in making the best decision for, and with, trafficked persons.

Imagine two different scenarios:

A 14-year-old girl is referred to you with symptoms of PTSD. After
fully informing your patient of any reporting requirements you have
in your jurisdiction, she tells you that the traumatic events that she
is struggling with include being forced by her boyfriend to have sex
with more than 20 men a day. Your patient tells you that she is a runaway and has been living with her boyfriend for more than a year.

In a second scenario, a 31-year-old presents with symptoms of depression, including suicidal ideation. She is struggling with feelings
of shame because, she says, she sells her body for sex. Upon further
discussion, your patient informs you that her "pimp" forces her to sell
sex so that she and her child have a place to live and that he keeps
all the money that she makes.

Can a physician do more than render medical treatment in situations like these? Are clinicians required, or allowed, to report anything to law enforcement? How can clinicians advocate for their patients and assist the trafficked person in advocating for themselves?

These questions can be confusing because many states have different requirements. To begin with, the Health Insurance Portability and Accountability Act of 1996 (P.L. 104-191), also known as HIPAA, outlines the requirements for health care providers in keeping patient information confidential. This law also outlines explicit circumstances in which confidential information may be disclosed. States have varied reporting requirements, but there are some general trends among them. If clinicians are unsure whether their state allows or requires reporting of instances of trafficking, they should check with the legal counsel for their place of employment. Finally, even if practitioners are not able to disclose confidential patient information, they may give the trafficked person resources and advocate for trafficked persons in a more general sense through legislative advocacy or volunteering at other organizations.

DISCLOSURE OF PATIENT STATUS AND HIPAA

Health Insurance Portability and Accountability Act

HIPAA required the Secretary of Health and Human Services to publicize standards for the privacy of health information. The final regulation, entitled the Privacy Rule, was published on December 28, 2000, and modified in August 2002 (Standards for Privacy of Individually Identifiable Health Information, 2000, 2002).

HIPAA applies to most health care providers and organizations, referred to as "covered entities" by HIPAA. The Centers for Medicare and Medicaid Services provides an online tool for determining whether your position or facility falls under HIPPA requirements (Centers for Medicare and Medicare Services 2016). If you transmit health information electronically, you are likely a "covered entity" under HIPAA (U.S. Department of Health and Human Services 2003).

HIPAA protects certain "individually identifiable health information," also known as "protected health information." This protected information includes that which identifies, or that for which there is a reasonable basis to believe could be used to identify, the individual and relates to

- The individual's past, present, or future physical or mental health condition,
- The provision of health care to the individual, or
- The past, present, or future payment for the provision of health care to the individual.

This includes, but is not limited to, common identifiers like name, date of birth, and social security number.

There are limited exceptions to these requirements for any patient, including when the health care provider receives permission from the individual or under specific circumstances defined by HIPAA (Powell et al. 2017). Health care providers may disclose protected health information to law enforcement under six circumstances:

(1) as required by law (including court orders, court-ordered warrants, subpoenas) and administrative requests; (2) to identify or locate a suspect, fugitive, material witness, or missing person; (3) in response to a law enforcement official's request for information about a victim or suspected victim of a crime; (4) to alert law enforcement of a person's death, if the covered entity suspects that criminal activity caused the death; (5) when a covered entity believes that protected health information is evidence of a crime that occurred on its premises; and (6) by a covered health care provider in a medical emergency not occurring on its premises, when necessary to inform law enforcement about the commission and nature of a crime, the location of the crime or crime victims, and the perpetrator of the crime. (45 Code of Federal Regulations § 164.512[f] [2004])

These exceptions may seem confusing; however, boiled down, these are the exceptions that will most likely be relevant to clinicians: 1) if the law requires disclosure through a mandatory reporting requirement or a court order, 2) if law enforcement makes a request for information about a victim of a crime, or 3) if you know of a medical emergency occurring somewhere else.

If none of these exceptions apply, clinicians must get authorization from the trafficked person to disclose any of their protected health information, including health information related to their trafficking victimization. To obtain authorization from the trafficked person for use of their protected health information, clinicians must obtain specific, written authorization in plain language (45 Code of Federal Regulations § 164.508 [2018]). Authorization must include the following: 1) a description of the information to be used or disclosed that identifies the information in a specific and meaningful fashion, 2) the name or other specific identification of the person authorized to make the requested use or disclosure, 3) the name or other specific identification of the person to whom you may make the requested use or disclosure, 4) a description of each purpose of the requested use or disclosure, 5) an expiration date or event that relates to the individual or purpose of the use or disclosure, and 6) the signature of the individual and date. Additionally, the authorization must include notice of the individual's right to revoke in writing; the ability or inability to condition treatment, payment, or enrollment or eligibility for benefits on the authorization; and the potential for information disclosed pursuant to the authorization to be subject to redisclosure by the recipient of the information and no longer to be protected by HIPAA. Finally, the health care provider must maintain a copy of this authorization and give a copy to the individual.

Another important factor to consider with respect to trafficked children is whether or not the child's parents will have access to the records of their treatment. HIPAA generally allows parents or legal guardians to have access to the medical records of their minor dependents. There are three exceptions to this: 1) when the minor consents to the treatment and the consent of the parent is not required under state law, 2) when the minor obtains treatment at the direction of the court, and 3) when the parent agrees that the minor and the health care provider may have a confidential relationship (U.S. Department of Health and Human Services 2017). Many states allow minors to consent to treatment for sexual health and psychological services without the parent's consent, and, therefore, this information could remain undisclosed. However, these provisions are state specific. To determine what your state's requirements are, there are several avenues available to you. Clinicians can check with their facility's legal representation and supervisors first. Most states also provide guidance to practitioners through the Department of Human Services or a similar agency. Finally, the National Human Trafficking Hotline can also provide guidance.

Clinician Responsibility to Disclose

Are clinicians permitted or required to disclose their patients' status as victims of human trafficking and simultaneously comply with HIPAA? The answer, unfortunately, is complicated.

For the Minor Patient

For the 14-year-old patient in the first scenario at the beginning of this chapter, clinicians must first determine if their state includes sex trafficking in their mandatory child abuse reporting laws. If so, check to see if the state limits reporting requirements to acts committed by a perpetrator who is a parent, guardian, or custodian. Because your patient's trafficker is her "older boyfriend," you will only be able to disclose the abuse if the state does not limit reporting in this way. If you are required to report the trafficked person's status as a trafficking victim, HIPAA requires that clinicians disclose only what is required by law and not more.

If clinicians are required to report their patient's status as a trafficking victim, there are several steps they should take to ensure the best course of treatment for their patient. First, it is likely that the patient's parents (or legal guardian) will find out about her status as a trafficking victim. Talk at length with the trafficked person to explain the steps that will follow. Volunteer to help her inform her parents. Second, emphasize to the patient that she has not done anything wrong, that she did not deserve to be trafficked, and that it is not her fault. Finally, ask the trafficked person if she would like to be present when the disclosure is made to authorities.

Depending on your individual state's law, reporting might be made to child protective services or law enforcement. When possible, try to work with law enforcement and child protective services staff who have been trained specifically on trafficking. Many states have child advocacy centers with trained forensic interviewers and staff to help minimize retraumatization of victims who enter the criminal justice process. It is critical to conduct safety planning with your patient. Although clinicians are not mandated to report to the National Human Trafficking Hotline, it may be a helpful resource in identifying trained law enforcement and child protective services staff. The Hotline can also help clinicians refer the trafficked person to comprehensive medical, legal, psychiatric, and social services that are available in your jurisdiction. Confidentiality must still be protected when reporting to the National Human Trafficking Hotline unless you have the permission of the patient, but you can still provide general or hypothetical information to access resources for clinician and patient.

For the Adult Patient

For your adult patient discussed in the second scenario, most states do not require disclosure if she is a victim of trafficking, even under domestic abuse or elder abuse statutes. Many states that allow or require reporting of adult abuse to adult protective services require only reporting of "financial exploitation," so there is no specific protection for human trafficking (U.S. Department of Justice 2019). If you have a patient in this situation, you should check with your organization's legal counsel to determine if this type of exploitation is reportable in your state. If it is not reportable, that means you will have to obtain the trafficked person's permission to disclose protected health information. Follow the steps outlined in this section's discussion of HIPAA to ensure you are in compliance with the statute.

If you are not sure whether you are allowed to disclose the trafficked person's information, reach out to your facility's legal representation.

STATE REPORTING REQUIREMENTS

States have varying requirements when it comes to reporting human trafficking. Most states mandate reporting for child victims of sex trafficking, either under specific child abuse statutes as "sexual abuse" or separately defined as "sexual exploitation." Although not all states explicitly include trafficking in child abuse statutes, the definition of sexual abuse should cover instances of trafficking of children even if the states have not been proactive in explicitly including language relating to sexual exploitation of minors.

Existing child abuse and neglect laws typically include offenses such as "sexual abuse" or "sexual exploitation," which will encompass most sex trafficking cases involving minors as conduct that clinicians are required to report (Atkinson et al. 2016). However, because of the age of these statutes, they may not cover all instances of sex trafficking of minors. In some states, acts are reportable only if a parent, guardian, custodian, or person responsible for the child commits the acts (Atkinson et al. 2016). A few states, including Massachusetts, Pennsylvania, and California, have specific language in their reporting laws regarding human trafficking (Atkinson et al. 2016; Pennsylvania Child Protective Services Law, 23 PA Cons Stat § 6303 [2014]).

PATIENT AUTHORIZATION AND ADVOCACY

Authorization

If you do not receive authorization from your patient to report his or her trafficking victimization and you are not required to disclose it by law, does this mean that you cannot advocate for him or her?

No! There are still other steps clinicians can take to advocate for trafficked persons and to assist them in advocating for themselves.

Check to see if your employer has a protocol or organizational policy for screening and providing resources for victims of trafficking. Even if clinicians cannot disclose the trafficked person's protected health information, you can still call the National Human Trafficking Hotline. Clinicians may disclose nonidentifying information to the Hotline and ask hypothetical questions. The Hotline can also help provide clinicians with screening questions to determine if their patient is a victim of trafficking. Importantly, the Hotline can also direct clinicians to resources for the trafficked person.

Clinicians should provide the trafficked person with the National Human Trafficking Hotline number. The hotline is accessible 24 hours a day, 7 days a week, 365 days a year. Help is offered in over 200 languages, and it can be accessed by text message by texting 233733 or calling 888-373-7888. The hotline can provide your patient with resources such as housing services, substance use treatment, legal services, and more. Make sure to inform your patient that he or she may remain anonymous when contacting the hotline. If you live in a jurisdiction with a human trafficking task force or response team, there is typically a medical provider who is a member of the team. They should also be able to help point clinicians to location-specific resources.

Make it clear that the health care setting is a safe place for the trafficked person to return. Be up-front about any potential reporting requirements you have and about the confidentiality of the trafficked person's information. If you have a multidisciplinary practice, bring in a social worker and other resources to get the help your patient needs. It is also a good idea to have resources on hand to provide to your patients, so that in case they want help, they know where to turn.

Make sure to support the trafficked person in a trauma-informed manner so that the trafficked person feels safe talking to you and seeking help. A trauma-informed approach recognizes the physical, social, and emotional impact of trauma on the individual and incorporates victim-centered practices that make him or her feel more comfortable (Office for Victims of Crime, Training and Technical Assistance Center 2019). For example, it will probably take time before the trafficked person feels comfortable seeking additional help. Be patient and treat the trafficked person for any underlying medical issues. Legal and other professional services are difficult to provide if a victim is not ready to pursue them. Help your patients become confident about seeking other resources and help them plan for what they might encounter.

When an individual becomes involved with the criminal justice system, they may be easily retraumatized. This is especially true if the person feels he or she lacks control; feels threatened, vulnerable, or ashamed; or experiences unexpected changes. To help the trafficked person mitigate these feelings, use the Hotline to find law enforcement officers and other professionals who have been trained in trauma-informed approaches. Request that your patient have the choice about when meetings will take place and who will conduct the interview. The more control and safety that can be offered to the trafficked person, the more cooperative he or she will be and the less retraumatization she will experience.

If the trafficked person decides to seek legal assistance (for expunging or vacating criminal convictions or for prosecuting their trafficker), there are several things that he or she should expect. First, the trafficked person will have to recount his or her story multiple times. This by itself can be very traumatizing. It is important to find an attorney who is trained in trauma-informed lawyering skills to assist your patient. The American Bar Association can help connect clinicians with attorneys who have been trained to offer legal assistance to trafficking survivors (www.americanbar.org/groups/domestic_violence/survivor-reentry-project).

Advocacy

After clinicians have done all of this for their individual patient, there are still ways that they can be an advocate without violating HIPAA. Get involved—find organizations in your area that assist victims of trafficking and volunteer (National Human Trafficking Hotline 2019). Create more awareness by including flyers and resources for victims of trafficking in a visible space in your practice (National Human Trafficking Hotline 2019). Contact your legislators and encourage them to prioritize legislation that assists victims of trafficking, such as safe harbor and vacatur laws. (Rhodes 2015). *Vacatur* is a judicial ruling that sets aside a conviction. This legal remedy can be incredibly meaningful to trafficked persons who are trying to find housing and employment after exiting their trafficking situation.

CONCLUSION

The legal requirements for reporting instances of human trafficking can be confusing because they often vary from state to state. However, you can always use the National Human Trafficking Hotline to search for resources in your state without disclosing any protected patient information. The main things to remember are to be up-front with your patients about the potential requirement of reporting the trafficking and about what information will be protected. No matter what your reporting requirements, you should offer the trafficked person resources for comprehensive exit services. This may include connection with organizations that offer trauma therapy, drug and alcohol treatment, case management, and assistance finding housing and employment.

Feel free to distribute the following flowchart (Figure 13–1) depicting disclosure of patient information within your practice or to post it in a place that it will be easily accessible for reference.

Pearls and Pointers

- Be up-front with your patient about any reporting requirements and confidentiality.

- If your patient discloses that they have been trafficked, check to see if you have mandatory reporting requirements.

- Offer your patient resources, including the National Human Trafficking Hotline number.

- Advocate for your patients with your legislators and by volunteering at anti-trafficking organizations.

REFERENCES

45 Code of Federal Regulations § 164.512(f). October 1, 2004. Available at: www.law.cornell.edu/cfr/text/45/164.512. Accessed November 7, 2019.
45 Code of Federal Regulations § 164.508. October 1, 2018. Available at: www.law.cornell.edu/cfr/text/45/164.508. Accessed November 7, 2019.
Atkinson HG, Curnin KJ, Hanson NC: U.S. state laws addressing human trafficking: education of and mandatory reporting by health care providers and other professionals. Journal of Human Trafficking 2(2):111–138, 2016
Centers for Medicare and Medicare Services: Are you a covered entity? June 21, 2016. Available at: www.cms.gov/Regulations-and-Guidance/Administrative-Simplification/HIPAA-ACA/AreYouaCoveredEntity.html. Accessed November 7, 2019.
Health Insurance Portability and Accountability Act of 1996, Pub. L. No. 104-191, § 261-264

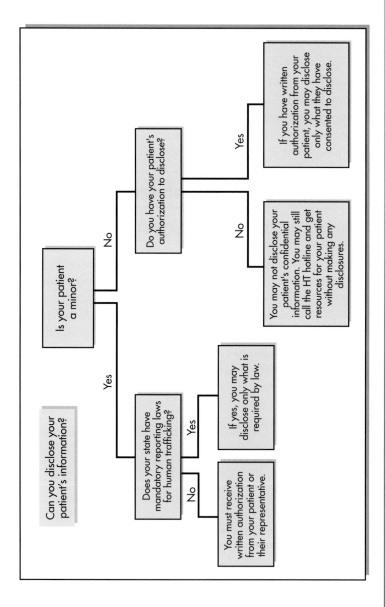

FIGURE 13–1. Decision making for disclosure of patient information.

National Human Trafficking Hotline: Get involved. 2019. Available at: https://humantraffickinghotline.org/get-involved. Accessed November 7, 2019.

Office for Victims of Crime, Training and Technical Assistance Center: Human Trafficking Task Force e-Guide: using a trauma-inform. 2019. Available at: www.ovcttac.gov/taskforceguide/eguide/4-supporting-victims/44-comprehensive-victim-services/mental-health-needs/substance-abuse-needs/. Accessed November 7, 2019.

Standards for Privacy of Individually Identifiable Health Information, 65 Fed. Register 82462. 2000

Standards for Privacy of Individually Identifiable Health Information, 67 Fed. Register 53182. 2002

Pennsylvania Child Protective Services Law, 23 PA Cons Stat § 6303 (2014). Available at: https://law.justia.com/codes/pennsylvania/2014/title-23/chapter-63/section-6303/. Accessed November 7, 2019.

Powell C, Asbill M, Brew S, et al: Human trafficking and HIPAA: what the health care professional needs to know. Journal of Human Trafficking 4(2):105–113, 2017

Rhodes SM: Why "safe harbor" full immunity is the best policy for decriminalizing child victims of sex trafficking. July 1, 2015. Available at: http://cseinstitute.org/wp-content/uploads/2015/06/Policy-Paper-Why-%E2%80%9CSafe-Harbor%E2%80%9D-Full-Immunity-is-the-Best-Policy-for-Decriminalizing-Child-Victims-of-Sex-Trafficking-.pdf. Accessed November 7, 2019.

U.S. Department of Health and Human Services: Summary of the HIPAA privacy rule. May 2003. Available at: www.hhs.gov/sites/default/files/privacysummary.pdf. Accessed November 7, 2019.

U.S. Department of Health and Human Services: Does the HIPAA privacy rule allow parents the right to see their children's medical records? Office of Civil Rights, October 17, 2017. Available at: www.hhs.gov/hipaa/for-professionals/faq/227/can-i-access-medical-record-if-i-have-power-of-attorney/index.html. Accessed November 7, 2019.

U.S. Department of Justice: Elder abuse and elder financial exploitation statutes. 2019. Available at: www.justice.gov/elderjustice/prosecutors/statutes?field_statute_state=MDandfield_statute_category=All. Accessed November 7, 2019.

CHAPTER 14

Survivor Voices

CASE SCENARIOS OF LABOR AND SEX TRAFFICKING

Holly Austin Gibbs, B.A.

Makini Chisolm-Straker, M.D., M.P.H.

> What would have worked most is if someone took the time to ask me any questions.
>
> *Barbara Amaya, author of* Nobody's Girl: A Memoir of Lost Innocence, Modern Day Slavery and Transformation *(2015)*

Human trafficking (aka, *trafficking in persons*) is a global issue. Every country is affected, including the United States. In 2000, the United States passed the Trafficking Victims Protection Act (TVPA; P.L. 106-386), which defines and outlaws two common forms of human trafficking: labor trafficking and sex trafficking. The TVPA's definition of human trafficking can be broken down into three parts: an action, a means, and a purpose (see Figure 14–1). At least one element from each part must be present in order to meet the federal definition of human trafficking (except in cases involving people less than 18 years of age, induced to perform commercial sex).

In partnership with HEAL Trafficking and Pacific Survivor Center, Dignity Health, a member of CommonSpirit Health, developed the PEARR Tool to help guide social workers, nurses, physicians, and other health care professionals on how to provide assistance to survivors of abuse, neglect, or violence, including human trafficking, in a trauma-informed manner. PEARR stands for the following steps: **P**rovide privacy, **E**ducate, **A**sk, **R**espect, and **R**espond. To learn

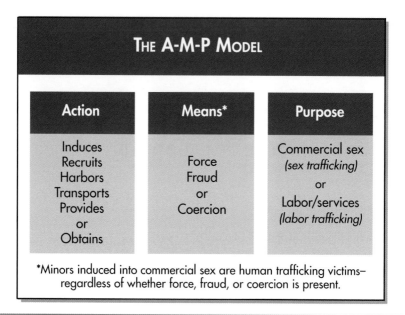

FIGURE 14–1. Action-Means-Purpose (A-M-P) model.

Commercial sex is defined by the Trafficking Victims Protection Act of 2000 as any sex act on account of which anything of value is given to or received by any person (e.g., money, drugs, survival needs).

Source. Reprinted from "Polaris: The Action Means Purpose "A-M-P" Model." 2012. Available at: https://traffickingresourcecenter.org/sites/default/files/AMP%20Model.pdf. Copyright © 2012 Polaris. Used with permission.

more about the PEARR Tool, see Chapter 8, "Responding to Human Trafficking in Health Care Settings."

In the following case scenarios, we learn more about how a human trafficking survivor might present in a health care setting. The questions provided are prompts for health care professionals learning how to use the PEARR Tool.

CASE 1

A young white girl presents to the emergency department (ED) late at night with jaundice. She appears younger than her stated age of 18. She complains of fatigue, poor appetite, stomach pain, fever, and nausea. You are concerned she is using drugs and is possibly homeless. The patient reports using heroin and needles. You offer to contact her family members; however, she states she has no family. She seems sad, extremely anxious, and exhausted.

Considering her confirmed substance use and given her potential homelessness, you are concerned the patient may be trading sex for survival needs.

Questions

1. Do you see possible red flags that put human trafficking on the differential? If yes, what are they?
   - The patient appears younger than stated age.
   - The patient feels a sense of familial abandonment, is homeless, and using illicit drugs.

2. Should you document the red flag(s)? What are your next steps?
   - Forensic documentation should be performed by clinicians trained in this skill because of the implications of how the medical record may be used in the patient's future (Shandro et al. 2016).
   - All clinically relevant documentation should occur as is necessary for the care of the patient. It is important to leave out "details" such as names and dates of events unless the documenter has been forensically trained; these details are not relevant or necessary to clinical care and can damage a patient's case in court (if the patient ever chooses to proceed to criminal or civil court).
   - New ICD-10 codes for human trafficking have recently been introduced. The use of "sensitive" diagnoses and terms such as "human trafficking" should be discussed with patients first; such diagnoses that may appear on discharge or billing paperwork should be included in safety planning discussions with patients. Clinicians should respect patient wishes here, in the interest of protecting their safety.

3. If the patient discloses that she is voluntarily trading sex for money, are you required to call law enforcement? If the patient requests or accepts help, how will you respond?
   - Under federal law, anyone less than 18 years of age engaged in any kind of commercial sex activity (including "prostitution," dancing in a strip club, and child abuse imagery) is considered a survivor of sex trafficking (Victims of Trafficking Victims Protection Act of 2000; P.L. 106-386). Clinicians are mandated reporters for concerns of labor and/or sex trafficking under the revised Child Abuse Prevention and Treatment

Act (P.L. 155-271) (see individual state laws indicating where such reports must be made [Atkinson et al. 2016]). Pediatric patients should be made aware that a report must be made (reports should not be made in secret, as this violates the trust of patients), but clinical care and patient safety should always come first.

- Clinicians are *not* mandated reporters for concerns of trafficking for adult (18 years and older) patients—unless the patient presents in a manner that is consistent with other mandated reporting requirements (e.g., in Arizona, if a physician, surgeon, nurse, or hospital attendant is called on to treat a person for gunshot wounds, knife wounds, or other material injuries that may have resulted from a fight, brawl, robbery, or other illegal or unlawful act, then that health care professional shall immediately notify the chief of police, city marshal, sheriff, or the nearest police officer of the circumstances, along with the name and description of the patient, the character of the wound, and other facts that may be of assistance to authorities in the event the condition of the patient may be due to any illegal transaction or circumstances; https://azleg.gov/ars/13/03806.htm).
- Unless mandated reporting applies, identifying information cannot be shared with anyone without patient consent as this is a violation of the Health Insurance Portability and Accountability Act (HIPAA) and could seriously endanger the safety of the patient. In this scenario and without more information, the clinician may not be mandated to report (see individual state laws).
- All patients should receive appropriate clinical care, regardless of reports made to any authoritative bodies. Institutions and practices should develop trauma-informed, patient-centered protocols that employ harm-reduction techniques to meet the social needs (e.g., drug detoxification/rehabilitation, shelter, legal assistance) of patients (HEAL Trafficking 2019).

Barbara Amaya's Story

Case 1 is based on an experience shared by Barbara Amaya, author of *Nobody's Girl: A Memoir of Lost Innocence, Modern Day Slavery, and Transformation*. In her memoir, Barbara describes years under the control of a violent "pimp" who was her trafficker.[1]

As a child, Barbara was sexually abused by a family member. Consequently, she began running away at a very early age. Ultimately, she was taken in by a couple who instructed her to exchange sex for money and who then sold her to a "pimp." Barbara spent her entire adolescence under the control of this violent "pimp" in New York City.

Barbara was 15 years old when she presented to the ED in the above scenario. She used heroin as a coping mechanism (not because she had been forced to do so by traffickers).[2] Today, Barbara is a nationally known speaker, subject matter expert, and consultant.

If Someone Took the Time...

Barbara says there is no one question that would have worked for her that night in the ED. Any number of questions might have worked. She was so tired that she just wanted someone to take care of her. What would have worked best for her, she says, is if someone took the time to ask her *any* questions; if someone took the time to show her compassion and genuine concern for her safety and well-being.

Barbara was not recognized as a victim that night. But she was grateful to have just been allowed to sleep in the ED for a few hours before returning to the streets.[3]

Learn more about Barbara Amaya at the website http://barbaraamaya.com/index.html.

CASE 2

A 14-year-old black girl presents to the ED with a broken knee; a bone is protruding from the open wound on her knee. Her mother states that they recently moved to the United States from Cameroon. The mother answers all questions and says her daughter fell while running. Her daughter fails to make eye contact and appears afraid.

---

[1]Telephone interview with Barbara Amaya by Holly Gibbs, Patient Care Services Program Director, Violence and Human Trafficking Prevention and Response Program, CommonSpirit Health, Summer 2015.

[2]Some data indicate that gang traffickers more commonly force drug use among their victims than do pimp traffickers (Smith 2014, p. 123).

[3]Telephone interview with Barbara Amaya by Holly Gibbs, Patient Care Services Program Director, Violence and Human Trafficking Prevention and Response Program, CommonSpirit Health, Summer 2015.

Questions

1. Is this child a potential victim of abuse?

   - The injury is more severe than expected based on the offered mechanism of injury. Child maltreatment is on the differential, as is underlying medical pathology.

2. Or is the child's behavior part of her culture?

   - Clinicians must be respectful of cultures to which they do not belong, but they cannot be experts in all the world's cultures. Clinicians should learn about the communities that they serve and become familiar with the behaviors, needs, and expectations of their patients (Office of Minority Health 2019). Many demeanors and behaviors, including apparent hostility, failure to make eye contact, and apparent timidity can be signs of abuse or trauma; they can also be signs of depression, anxiety, or fear of health practitioners, for example. This patient's behavior is concerning, based on Western expectations of social interaction.

3. What if the mother refuses to leave the patient's side when requested? Is this normal behavior or a red flag?

   - The patient is old enough to speak with a clinician privately. The mother's behavior is concerning for maltreatment or trauma, but some guardians are just extremely protective or want to be completely involved in the care of their child. It is important to approach each patient, and their visitors, respectfully and honestly. It can be helpful to refer to a generalized practice. For example, a clinician might say, "I know it is important to you that your daughter gets the best care possible. To do that, it is our practice to examine all adolescents [or patients] in a private space; thank you for helping us to provide the best care for your child. I'll come get you just as soon as the exam is complete, so we can all talk together." For the safety of the patient, it is important not to alienate the visitor; it should be made clear that privacy is an institutional practice, not the result of a patient's personal request or due to a specific suspicion.

Evelyn Chumbow's Story

Case 2 is based on Evelyn Chumbow's experience.[4] Evelyn was born in Cameroon and sold into slavery by her uncle. He visited Evelyn's village and told her mother that he could provide Evelyn with an education in the United States.

From the ages of 9 to 17 years, Evelyn worked as a domestic servant in a suburb of Maryland. She cooked, cleaned, and cared for her trafficker's children. She slept on the floor and was beaten for any perceived disobedience.

Both the uncle and the woman claiming to be Evelyn's mother are guilty of human trafficking under the TVPA. The uncle provided Evelyn as a domestic servant, and the woman obtained her.

Look Beneath the Surface

Evelyn was repeatedly assaulted by the woman claiming to be her mother. Evelyn wasn't recognized as a possible victim during this presentation; she was treated in the ED and discharged.

Evelyn's case is only one example that illustrates the importance of looking beneath the surface. Clinicians should be respectful but should not assume a patient's submissive demeanor is due to their[5] culture. Every mature patient with capacity *should be afforded time alone with their clinician (who should use certified medical interpreters when needed); even if abuse or exploitation is not suspected, this is an opportunity for the patient to disclose despite the clinician's lack of suspicion.* Evelyn says that had she been able to speak with a clinician alone, she would have answered questions honestly: she would have disclosed the abuse and exploitation she was experiencing.

After 8 years of domestic servitude, Evelyn ran away. Eventually, her case was handled by Homeland Security, and the abusive woman was arrested and convicted of human trafficking.[6]

---

[4]Telephone interview with Evelyn Chumbow by Holly Gibbs, Patient Care Services Program Director, Violence and Human Trafficking Prevention and Response Program, CommonSpirit Health, Summer 2015.
[5]The authors are purposefully forgoing traditional grammar rules to be inclusive of all people that can experience trafficking. People with a transgender or gender nonconforming life experience are often recognized as particularly vulnerable to being trafficked. The use of "they/their" in lieu of "s/he" is meant to be inclusive of all genders that experience human trafficking.
[6]Telephone interview with Evelyn Chumbow by Holly Gibbs, Patient Care Services Program Director, Violence and Human Trafficking Prevention and Response Program, CommonSpirit Health, Summer 2015.

Today, Evelyn is a wife, a mother, and an international advocate for people who have been trafficked. She graduated from college with a degree in homeland security and has served on the U.S. White House Advisory Council on Human Trafficking.

CASE 3

A 31-year-old biracial (black and white) woman presents to the ED with a 29-year-old white female companion. The patient has valid forms of identification and health insurance through state disability. The patient's finger is swelling; as a result, she is unable to remove a ring. The companion states the two of them had a fight, which is why the patient's hand appears to be bruised. You notice the patient is much taller and heavier—approximately 5 inches taller and 80 pounds heavier—than the companion. Both women appear to be timid, and they both fail to make eye contact with male nurses. The patient insists that she does not want to press charges against her friend.

Questions

1. During treatment, you notice a tattoo on the patient's chest—it depicts a man's name and dollar signs. Is this patient a potential victim of trafficking?

   - Tattoos can be brands, the way that a trafficker marks a person as their "property." It is not always obvious which tattoos are brands and which were desired. Rather than assign value to a tattoo, clinicians can simply ask, "Can you tell me about your tattoo?"

2. The fire department arrives to cut the ring from the patient's finger. During the process, you notice the patient winces in pain when one of the firefighters touches her back. How will you approach this patient about potential abuse? What if she chooses not to accept help?

   - All patients should be approached respectfully and with genuine concern for their safety, health, and well-being. See the PEARR Tool (available at the Dignity Health website: www.dignityhealth.org/human-trafficking-response) for additional guidance.
   - Depending on the state, clinicians may be mandated reporters of certain wounds and injuries, regardless of the age and ca-

pacity of the patient. On the basis of the history of the present illness (HPI) provided in Case 3, however, this may not be a situation in which a clinician would be a mandated reporter. (For example, in Nevada, health care providers are required to report to law enforcement only those injuries that appear to have been inflicted by means of a firearm or knife, not under accidental circumstances [State of Nevada 1977]; certain burns must also be reported to a local fire department [State of Nevada 1991]. See your individual state laws for details.)

- Clinicians must be familiar with their state laws so they can accurately describe their reporting requirements to patients. The mandated reporting principles discussed in Case 1 should be followed here too. Clinicians should explicitly state that the patient is welcome to return for clinical care in the future or for assistance in seeking safety. See the PEARR Tool for additional guidance.
- Although this patient does not want to file a police report, she may have other needs. A harm reduction approach requires that someone on the care team invite the patient to discuss other areas in which she may be interested in seeking assistance (Stratton et al. 2001).

3. Should you also approach the companion?

- The companion is not your patient. Talking to them about your patient, without your patient's permission, is a HIPAA violation.

Wendy Barnes' Story

Case 3 is based on an experience shared by Wendy Barnes, a survivor of sex trafficking. Wendy was trafficked by a violent "pimp" for more than 10 years. In this scenario, Wendy was the companion.[7]

The "pimp" in this case forced the patient and companion to lie about having a fight; this was the only way he would allow the patient to seek medical treatment after he brutally beat her. Wendy and the other women and girls under his control were often seen as criminals, or they were not "seen" at all.

---

[7]Email correspondence between Wendy Barnes and Holly Gibbs, Patient Care Services Program Director, Violence and Human Trafficking Prevention and Response Program, CommonSpirit Health, Summer 2015.

In her memoir, *And Life Continues: Sex Trafficking and My Journey to Freedom* (Barnes 2015), Wendy describes how she was trafficked for commercial sex by this man and how she finally regained her freedom. The "pimp," who was her trafficker, was ultimately sentenced to life in prison. Today, Wendy is the Patient Care Services Coordinator of CommonSpirit Health's Violence and Human Trafficking Prevention and Response Program.

If You Suspect a Companion Is a Victim of Trafficking...

Please keep in mind that the National Human Trafficking Hotline (https://humantraffickinghotline.org/) is available 24 hours a day, 7 days a week to do the following:

- Receive reports (anonymously, if desired) of suspicious activity or potential/certain cases of human trafficking in the community
- Provide information about local resources available to trafficked persons, as well as local organizations working on awareness and prevention
- Support staff when caring for potential/actual patients victimized by trafficking
- Speak via telephone with patients about possible victimization and connect trafficked persons with local/national resources according to the patient's wishes

The National Human Trafficking Hotline allows callers to report suspicious activity and learn about local and national resources; it provides real-time assistance to clinical staff and/or patients. Hotline specialists speak both English and Spanish and can communicate with callers in 200+ additional languages by using a telephone interpreting service.

CASE 4

A 19-year-old Southeast Asian woman presents to the ED late Saturday night with an Asian American man in his late 30s. The patient has a large bruise and a cut on her forehead that requires sutures. The man says the patient is a family friend who lives with him and his wife, and she fell in the yard.

He says the patient does not speak English and insists on answering questions on her behalf. The patient agrees to allow the man to speak on her behalf; however, she appears to be afraid.

Questions

1. Once alone with the patient, what might you say?

   - If you do not share a language in common, always use a certified medical interpreter (Office of Minority Health 2019). These professionals are trained on confidentiality principles, relevant clinical terminology, and the best techniques to foster the patient-practitioner bond that would naturally develop when the patient and clinician speak the same language.
   - Start at the beginning. Tell the patient she is not in trouble with you; rather, explain that it is institutional practice to speak with all patients privately and to use certified medical interpreters when necessary.
   - Ask her about why she came to the health care facility. This allows her to tell about more than the injury that is apparent. If the HPI does not correlate with the injury, respectfully explain why you do not understand what happened. If she insists on the previously offered mechanism, tell her that you are going to help take care of her injury and you also believe she may be in trouble. Let her know you would like to connect her with available services if she is interested now or at another time. Remind her that nothing you discuss can be discussed with her employer without her permission (be honest about mandated reporting laws whenever applicable).

2. The patient says she works more than 12 hours a day with little pay but she believes she is bound by a contract. Is there a way to inform her of her rights as an immigrant worker?

   - Without knowing the details of her employment contract and unless the clinician also has expertise in this area, it is best not to offer legal advice. Rather, clinicians can offer sympathy for the long hours and offer to connect the patient with local resources to help determine if her rights are being respected.
   - The U.S. Department of State has created a video and pamphlet to explain rights, protections, and resources available to temporary employees in the United States. The pamphlets are available in multiple languages and can be printed from the Department of State website (U.S. Department of State 2019).

The U.S. Department of Labor also has resources available to provide workers with basic information to recognize situations of labor exploitation (www.dol.gov/agencies/whd/resources/videos/know-your-rights).

3. The patient shares that the man's wife assaulted her; she asks for help. The local resource for assault victims will not be able to respond until the morning. Do you keep the patient overnight?

    - Clinical care should always come first. If the patient requires admission for medical or psychiatric care, you should admit or transfer them, as necessary.
    - If the patient is clinically safe for discharge, and wants to leave her situation, and needs a safe place to stay, you should work within your power to arrange that. A previously designed protocol should identify resources that can be called on; if shelter/housing is not available at the time, determine when it may become available. It may be feasible to have the patient wait a few hours in the ED or in the observation unit, for example, until a bed is available. Depending on institutional practice and resources, a patient may be able to stay at the health care facility longer.

Ima Matul's Story

Case 4 is based on an experience shared by Ima Matul.[8] Ima was lured to the United States from Indonesia with a false job promise and forced into domestic servitude in a Los Angeles, California, suburb.

On this particular day, Ima had been assaulted by one of her employers, the man's wife. Ima says that had she been separated from the man and approached in the right way, she would have answered clinicians' questions honestly and accepted help. Unfortunately, the man was allowed to interpret on Ima's behalf, and Ima was not recognized as a trafficked person. Ima later escaped the home and received assistance from the Coalition to Abolish Slavery and Trafficking.

Today, Ima Matul is an international advocate for trafficked persons. She oversees the National Survivor Network, a program created by the Coalition to Abolish Slavery and Trafficking in Los

---

[8]In-person interview with Ima Matul by Holly Gibbs, Patient Care Services Program Director, Violence and Human Trafficking Prevention and Response Program, CommonSpirit Health, and email correspondence, Summer 2015.

Angeles, California. In 2012, Ima was recognized by President Barack Obama at the Clinton Global Initiative.

CASE 5

A 14-year-old white boy presents to the ED alone, late at night, complaining of an injury to his rectum after falling off his bicycle. He appears dirty and disheveled. He smells of alcohol, and he appears anxious, angry, and seems very distrustful of staff. He produces identification that lists his home address in a different county.

Questions

1. How would you respond to the patient's irritability and obvious lack of trust in medical staff or other authorities?
2. Examination findings of rectal trauma make the clinician concerned for sexual assault. Are you required to call child welfare and/or law enforcement?

   • If the HPI is not consistent with the mechanism of injury and the clinician is concerned for child maltreatment, the clinician is a mandated reporter. But clinical care and safety must always come first; clinicians should be honest with patients about their requirements as mandated reporters, and clinicians do not have the authority to detain patients.

3. Do you tell the patient that you are calling authorities? Knowing the patient may leave against medical advice once he is informed, what are some ways to provide trauma-informed care to this patient?

   • Clinicians should always be honest about mandated reporting requirements. Clinicians should also emphasize the care team's priority is safely providing high-quality health care. Ask the patient about their goals and offer to meet those needs before making the report. If reporting is required,[9] offer to make the report together, so they know what is shared. Clini-

---

[9]According to the amended Child Abuse Prevention and Treatment Act (P.L. 155-271), "child abuse and neglect" is defined as, "at a minimum, any recent act or failure to act on the part of a parent or caretaker which results in death, serious physical or emotional harm, sexual abuse or exploitation" or as "an act or failure to act which presents an imminent risk of serious harm."

cians do not have the authority to detain patients with capacity. If patients are afraid to seek health care because of clandestine mandated reporting, their health will suffer.

4. How might you build rapport with this patient?

- Ask him about his goals of care; why did he come to the health care facility?
- Demonstrate genuine concern and respect. Let him know that he can refuse any part of the exam and that he does not have to answer questions that make him uncomfortable.
- Offer him food and drink if that is available.
- Be honest. Do not make promises you cannot keep; do not make threats. Make the rules of engagement clear—explain what behavior is acceptable in the health care facility.

5. What resources might you offer this patient, especially if the patient is a flight risk?

- Based on what he tells you he needs, offer him connection to or information about resources. If you have the capacity to provide what he needs, offer to do so.
- Based on your professional expertise, offer other connections or information too. If you have the capacity to provide what he needs, offer to do so.

  Have this conversation before you complete your first encounter in case he elopes.

Greg Bucceroni's Story

Case 5 is based on an experience shared by Greg Bucceroni,[10] a survivor of childhood sexual abuse and sex trafficking (Smith 2014, p. 37). Greg was sexually exploited commercially in three states with other teenage boys, many of whom were homeless and selling sex to survive on the streets. He says he often visited EDs, mostly because of physical altercations with other youth and with adult criminals.

On this particular night, Greg was at a hotel party hosted by men who were exploiting Greg and his friends. Another man joined the party—someone that Greg did not know—and this man ultimately

---

[10]Telephone interview with Greg Bucceroni by Holly Gibbs, Patient Care Services Program Director, Violence and Human Trafficking Prevention and Response Program, CommonSpirit Health, and email correspondence, Summer 2015.

drugged and raped Greg that night. After being interviewed in the ED, Greg was told that his parents had to be contacted. He suspected staff had also called police, so he quietly eloped.

Today, Greg Bucceroni is an outspoken activist against child sex predators and an advocate for runaway/homeless youth and male survivors of sexual abuse and sex trafficking. He currently works as a community support specialist for Town Watch Integrated Services in Philadelphia, Pennsylvania.

Interviewing Youth and Young Adults

Young patients, especially runaway or homeless teenagers, may be distrustful of authorities, often with good reason (Bigelsen and Vuotto 2013; Love et al. 2018; Young Women's Empowerment Project 2009). In a video titled *Uncovering the Truth: Identifying Sexually Exploited Youth in a Health Setting*,[11] a group of young survivors offer advice to health professionals. One survivor recommends asking open-ended questions. A clinician might say something like the following:

> I know it's hard for those surviving on the streets. Sometimes people can get caught up in "the life" or in a way of life in which they're forced to trade sex to survive. If you or someone you know needs help, please know this is a safe place, there are resources available, and you can talk to me. Can you tell me about (your injury, home life, needs)?

When working with runaway and homeless youth, asking open-ended questions is the most efficacious way to learn how clinicians can help and to figure out what available resources might be useful. The National Runaway Safeline also offers free downloadable brochures (available at www.1800runaway.org/free-promotional-materials). These may be helpful when discussing resources with patients. Their general brochure describes an overview of services available to runaway, homeless, and other youth at risk of being trafficked.

---

[11] *Uncovering the Truth: Identifying Sexually Exploited Youth in a Health Setting*, DVD, coproduced by Global Health Promise, End Child Prostitution and Sex Trafficking (ECPAT)-USA, Girls Educational and Mentoring Services (GEMS); for information on ordering the DVD, contact info@ecpatusa.org.

CASE 6

A 41-year-old South Asian man presents late at night, with his 37-year-old wife, to the ED via ambulance. He collapsed at home and his family called 911. The patient is sweating profusely and is extremely anxious, light-headed, and complaining of a bad headache. He denies use of cigarettes, alcohol, or other drugs.

During treatment, he and his wife seem anxious about producing documentation and paying for medical bills. The wife seems unsure of whom to call or where to turn. After several hours, the patient is admitted.

Questions

1. During the care course, the patient tells you that he is unemployed. He and his wife formerly worked for a local restaurant. They moved here from India to work for a family friend who owns the restaurant, but it seems the relationship ended poorly. The patient seems anxious about the former employer, but you are unsure why. Do you suspect labor exploitation or labor trafficking? What questions might you ask? Would you take any additional actions?

    - Focus on the clinical needs of the patient first.
    - Because of the Emergency Medical Treatment and Active Labor Act (part of the Consolidated Omnibus Budget Reconciliation Act of 1985; P.L. 99-272), EDs that accept Medicare and Medicaid must emergently evaluate and care for all patients, regardless of their ability to pay. Make the wife aware of this law, offer to connect her with the hospital social worker (if available) to discuss medical billing, and ask in what other ways she needs help. Ask her if it is okay to talk with a hospital social worker about her and her husband's nonclinical care-related needs, so they can access relevant and available services, including local resources for immigrant populations.

2. The patient shares that the former employer is harassing the patient. He says the employer took loans out in the patient's name and defaulted on the loans. The patient is stressed out because credit collectors are calling his home and threatening legal action against him. Are you required to contact law enforcement against the patient's wishes?

    - Even if you suspect trafficking, you cannot violate HIPAA. Unless the patient presents in a way that meets mandated reporting requirements, then you must have that patient's permission to share specific details of a trafficking concern with law enforcement. In this scenario, the clinical presentation may not warrant a report to any agency (see individual state laws).

Harold D'Souza's Story

Harold D'Souza was lured to the United States from India by a family friend, a man who promised Harold and his family a better life and opportunity. This man (the "employer") used falsified documents, however, and trapped Harold in a job with threats of incarceration and deportation.

Harold worked more than 14 hours per day and was never paid. The employer used Harold's information to open financial accounts. Harold escaped the employer but could not find other work. He was harassed, not only by the former employer but also by credit collectors. The D'Souzas did not know the law in the United States and did not know where to turn. After a hospitalization, Harold began a long journey navigating the U.S. legal system to become a documented immigrant. In the end, he and his family finally gained independence from his trafficker.[12]

Today, Harold and his wife, Dancy, are advocates for survivors of human trafficking. Harold currently serves on the U.S. Advisory Council on Human Trafficking. Learn more about Harold at the Eyes Open International website (www.eyesopeninternational.org).

Immigrants Are a Vulnerable Population

Immigrant workers, especially undocumented immigrants, can and often do become victims of crime.

- Any immigrant (regardless of documentation status) can be vulnerable to exploitation if lacking sufficient support or resources.
- Labor traffickers often target vulnerable immigrants with whom they can communicate and build trust and those with whom they share a similar ethnicity or background.

---

[12]Telephone interview with Harold D'Souza by Holly Gibbs, Patient Care Services Program Director, Violence and Human Trafficking Prevention and Response Program, CommonSpirit Health, and email correspondence, Summer 2015.

Be sure to connect vulnerable immigrant patients with local resources. Harold says he was not identified as a trafficked or exploited person during his hospital stay and that it would have been
helpful if he and his wife were seen by a social worker.[13]

CASE 7

A 19-year-old white woman presents to the ED in the custody of law
enforcement. She is shaking uncontrollably, covered in bruises, and
underweight, weighing about 84 pounds. Law enforcement arrested
the patient for prostitution but brought her to the ED for a medical
evaluation. They are seeking clearance to detain her in jail. Unable
to participate in history or exam because of the acuity of her presentation, the patient tests positive for opioid use and for pregnancy in
the course of her medical assessment.

Questions

1. Is this patient a potential victim of sex trafficking? Why or why not?

   - Anyone involved in the commercial sex industry can be at risk
     of sex trafficking. Traffickers often target young people work-
     ing in the commercial sex industry, whether it is illegal work
     (e.g., outdoor solicitation) or legal work (e.g., strip clubs, adult
     pornography).

2. How might the clinical team determine if the patient wants help
   (medical or otherwise)?

   - Ask the patient.

3. What if the patient reports being assaulted by a "pimp"? How
   would you respond?

   - Provide clinical care first. If, on the basis of the HPI provided,
     you are not a mandated reporter, ask her if she wants to speak
     with law enforcement about the assault. Respect her wishes.
     It is against the law to do otherwise.

4. What if the patient denies having been assaulted or controlled by
   a "pimp" but requests help?

---

[13]Telephone interview with Harold D'Souza by Holly Gibbs, Patient Care
Services Program Director, Violence and Human Trafficking Prevention and
Response Program, CommonSpirit Health, and email correspondence, Sum-
mer 2015.

- Specifically identify what help she wants, and then determine if you can help facilitate connections to relevant services. Decide, based on your professional training, if there are other services you think may also help her; offer those (and why you think they will be helpful) as well.

Christine "Clarity" McDonald's Story

Case 7 is based on an experience shared by Christine "Clarity" McDonald.[14] Christine ran away from home as a young teenager. She was found by a man and coerced into working as a dancer in a strip club, where she was introduced to and developed a chemical dependence on cocaine.

Because of the substance use disorder, Christine was unable to work consistently and lost her job. She was homeless and started using crack cocaine. Christine sold sex to survive and was trafficked by various "pimps" over several years. She was arrested 103 times. To learn more about Christine's story, read her memoir, *Cry Purple* (McDonald 2013). Christine has also published a book titled *The Same Kind of Human: Seeing the Marginalized and Exploited Through Eyes of Grace* (McDonald 2016).

Compassion and Dignity

During this particular hospital visit, Christine was under the control of a violent "pimp" and was severely malnourished. She was treated by law enforcement and medical staff as if she "was a disease." Christine emphasizes the importance of treating all patients with compassion and dignity.[15] Today, Christine is a mother, an author, and a national advocate for survivors of human trafficking and persons struggling with substance use disorders and homelessness. Her advocacy efforts have resulted in legislative changes in Missouri that help support persons convicted of felonies and trying to overcome substance use disorders and homelessness.

---

[14]Telephone interview with Christine McDonald by Holly Gibbs, Patient Care Services Program Director, Violence and Human Trafficking Prevention and Response Program, CommonSpirit Health, and email correspondence, Summer 2015.

[15]Telephone interview with Christine McDonald by Holly Gibbs, Patient Care Services Program Director, Violence and Human Trafficking Prevention and Response Program, CommonSpirit Health, and email correspondence, Summer 2015.

Learn more about Christine at the Christine's Vision website (www.christinesvision.org).

CASE 8

A young Southeast Asian woman presents to a clinic for a mandated tuberculosis test. She has recently entered the United States on a temporary visa to work in a nursing facility with elderly patients. The patient is accompanied by her employer, an older Southeast Asian woman who insists on answering questions on the patient's behalf. You notice the companion is holding the patient's identification and documents. When asked to wait outside, the companion stands near the door within ear shot. The patient seems shy.

Questions

1. Do you see red flags of human trafficking? What might you say to the patient or patient's companion?

   • By now, the reader is familiar with trafficking indicators and the appropriate actions to answer the following questions.

2. What are your next steps?
3. What if the companion refuses to leave the room? How will you respond?
4. What resources can you offer to this patient regarding her rights as a temporary worker in the United States?

Angela Guanzon's Story

Angela Guanzon was recruited from the Philippines to work in Los Angeles, California, in a nursing facility for elderly patients. The recruiters confiscated Angela's passport and work visa before she left Los Angeles International Airport. She was told she owed $12,000 for entry into the United States and that it would take 10 years to pay off the debt. Angela was not allowed to leave the nursing facility and was forced to sleep on the floor. After 2 years, Angela and other survivors were finally found by law enforcement.[16]

---

[16]In-person interview with Angela Guanzon by Holly Gibbs, Patient Care Services Program Director, Violence and Human Trafficking Prevention and Response Program, CommonSpirit Health, and email correspondence, Summer 2015.

Angela says that receiving information about her rights as a temporary worker in the United States would have helped her the most.

Angela Guanzon is now a medical biller and coder, a member of the National Survivor Network, and a former board member of HEAL Trafficking.

CASE 9

A 20-year-old white woman presents to a hospital labor and delivery floor in active labor. This is her second child. She is accompanied by a white woman who appears to be young (possibly under age 18) and a black man (patient's stated boyfriend and father of the baby). *The patient seems anxious and quiet.*

The young female companion comes and goes throughout the evening. You notice the patient's boyfriend is flirtatious with the nurses and with the female companion. In fact, you often see him outside of the patient's room with the female companion. In one of these encounters, you notice the man taking a large amount of cash from her.

Questions

1. Are there red flag(s) of human trafficking? What are your next steps?
2. Do you attempt to speak with the patient alone? If so, how will you separate the companion(s) from the patient?
3. When you are in a private area with the patient, what might you ask or say?
4. After delivery of the baby, a nurse notifies you that bruises were seen on the patient during delivery. Are you required to contact law enforcement? Adult protective services? Child welfare? If so, how will you inform the patient?

   - Some states require the reporting of certain wounds or injuries associated with intimate partner violence (IPV) or other forms of violence, regardless of the adult patient's desire to report (Kentucky Rev. Stat. Ann. 2008; N.M. Stat. Ann. 2008; California Penal Code 2008). If, after speaking with the patient, the clinician is concerned that the bruises are not reasonably related to another cause and may be the result of IPV or another kind of assault, the clinician may be a mandated reporter. To which authorities such reports must be made depends on the state. Clinicians must be familiar with the mandated reporting requirements of the states in which they practice. However, most states respect that an adult patient with capacity has the right to decline making an IPV report; that is, in most states IPV does not require a clinician report (clinicians must be up-to-date on their state's mandated reporting laws). Moreover, research demonstrates that people who experience IPV do not support mandated reporting or law enforcement intervention (Gielen et al. 2000, 2006; Glass et al. 2001; Rodríguez et al. 2001, 2002). There is concern, and some evidence, that patients' health and safety (or that of loved ones) may be endangered by mandated IPV reports, and some people may avoid needed clinical care to prevent clinician-initiated reports (Futures Without Violence 2019; Iyengar 2009).

- Patients should be made aware of the mandated report, ideally before the report is made. In fact, best practice includes telling a patient about the clinician's requirements as a mandated reporter before gathering information that may require (based on state law) a report.

Wendy Barnes' Story

Case 9 is based on another experience shared by Wendy Barnes, a survivor of sex trafficking mentioned in Case 3.[17] In this scenario, Wendy is the patient and the male companion is her trafficker. The female companion—a young teenager—is also being trafficked by the male companion. He forced the teenager to continue working on the street while Wendy was in the hospital. Wendy ultimately had three children with this man; at least one other trafficking survivor also had a child with him. This man was later sentenced to life in prison for sex trafficking of adults and minors.

Wendy says that if staff had been educated about sex trafficking and looking for red flags, it would have been obvious that this man was a "pimp" and that he was trafficking both Wendy and the girl. Wendy says that both she and the female companion appeared eager to please the man. Wendy also points out that the trafficker presented to staff as "charming"—not intimidating.

---

[17]In-person interview with Wendy Barnes by Holly Gibbs, Patient Care Services Program Director, Violence and Human Trafficking Prevention and Response Program, CommonSpirit Health, and email correspondence, Summer 2015.

Planting Seeds of Hope

As a child, Wendy had been sexually abused by her stepfather. Child welfare removed Wendy from the home, but Wendy's mother moved Wendy back in and told her to stay on the second floor (away from the stepfather). This was Wendy's foundation for and understanding of love, family, and home. Wendy's trafficker preyed on women and girls with backgrounds similar to Wendy's. Traffickers prey on vulnerability.

Day after day, this man told his victims they were worthless and that nobody would love them except him. What Wendy needed most, she says, was a counternarrative. Any time an outsider offered her compassion and respect, it was like planting a seed, a seed that ultimately bloomed into the strength she needed to fight back and to become the national advocate for survivors that she is today.

CASE 10

A 20-year-old black woman presents to a clinic; she is told she is 3 months pregnant. She seems sad but unsurprised. Although she returns for antenatal care, she often misses her appointments and has to reschedule. She is chronically anemic and frequently presents with dehydration and urinary tract infections.

When asked about her symptoms, the patient attributes them to being a single mother with a toddler at home. When asked about work and family, the patient seems evasive. Do you suspect abuse, neglect, or exploitation?

Questions

1. Are there red flag(s) of human trafficking?
2. What are your next steps?
3. If the patient shares that she trades sex for money, are you required to call law enforcement? Adult protective services? Child welfare?
4. If the patient admits to having a boyfriend who helps to schedule her "dates," are you required to call law enforcement? Adult protective services? Child welfare?
5. What resources can you recommend if she requests support/assistance?

Tanya Gould's Story

Case 10 is based on an experience shared by Tanya Gould, a survivor of sex trafficking and member of the U.S. White House Advisory Council on Human Trafficking. Tanya provided the following message for Dignity Health's educational module, *Human Trafficking 101: Dispelling the Myths* (available at https://webhost.dignity-health.org/elearning/launch.html?val=SFRSUDEwMQ==):

> I was trafficked at 18 until I was 21. During that time, I visited the emergency room at least 3 times for a UTI. I also had a baby and made multiple trips to our family doctor for shots and well visits. After a year, I became pregnant with a second child. The visits I made to the emergency rooms and doctors' offices were in my home town. Often, I think about those times and wonder how many medical providers wanted to reach out to me but didn't know how.
>
> Thank you for your commitment to identify and protect victims in your facility. Today I am a wife, a mother, and a college graduate.[18]

Tanya is the founder of Identifiable Me, a victim services organization in Virginia addressing gender-based violence. Learn more about Tanya at the Identifiable Me website (http://identifiableme.org).

CONCLUSION

Human trafficking is a heavy topic, and education on this topic can leave many learners feeling hopeless. However, with a trauma-informed approach to intervention and with connections to appropriate community agencies, people who are experiencing this type of victimization can overcome and even thrive. Barbara Amaya, Christine McDonald, and Wendy Barnes are all published authors; Evelyn Chumbow, Harold D'Souza, and Tanya Gould are all current or former members of the U.S. White House Advisory Council on Human Trafficking. Angela Guanzon currently works as a medical biller and coder, and Greg Bucceroni works as a community support specialist for Town Watch Integrated Services in Philadelphia, Pennsylvania. Like many survivors, Ima Matul is internationally known for her

---

[18]Email correspondence between Tanya Street and Holly Gibbs, Patient Care Services Program Director, Violence and Human Trafficking Prevention and Response Program, CommonSpirit Health, Summer 2015.

work against human trafficking; in 2012, she was recognized by President Barack Obama at the Clinton Global Initiative. In sharing the stories of survivors, the authors aspire to show that, with opportunity and capacity, there is space for hope.

REFERENCES

Amaya B: Nobody's Girl: A Memoir of Lost Innocence, Modern Day Slavery, and Transformation. Pittsburgh, PA, Animal Media Group, 2015

Atkinson HG, Curnin KJ, Hanson NC: U.S. state laws addressing human trafficking: education of and mandatory reporting by health care providers and other professionals. Journal of Human Trafficking 2(2):111–138, 2016

Barnes W: And Life Continues: Sex Trafficking and My Journey to Freedom. Scotts Valley, CA, CreateSpace Independent Publishing Platform, 2015

Bigelsen J, Vuotto S: Homelessness, Survival Sex, and Human Trafficking: As Experienced by the Youth of Covenant House. New York, Covenant House New York, 2013

California Penal Code § 11160 (West 2008)

Child Abuse Prevention and Treatment Act (as amended by P.L. 155-271), 132 STAT 3894, October 24, 2018.

Consolidated Omnibus Budget Reconciliation Act of 1985 (COBRA). Pub. L. No. 99-272, Title IX, Section 9121, 100 Stat 167 (1986)

Dignity Health: Human Trafficking 101: Dispelling the Myths. 2019. Available at: https://webhost.dignityhealth.org/elearning/launch.html?val=SFRSUDEwMQ==. Accessed November 10, 2019.

Futures Without Violence: Mandatory reporting of domestic violence to law enforcement by health care providers: a guide to advocates working to respond to or amend reporting laws related to domestic violence. 2019. Available at: www.futureswithoutviolence.org/userfiles/Mandatory_Reporting_of_DV_to_Law%20Enforcement_by_HCP.pdf. Accessed November 10, 2019.

Gielen AC, O'Campo PJ, Campbell JC, et al: Women's opinions about domestic violence screening and mandatory reporting. Am J Prev Med 19(4):279–285, 2000 11064232

Gielen AC, Campbell JC, Garza MA, et al: Domestic violence in the military: women's policy preferences and beliefs concerning routine screening and mandatory reporting. Military Medicine 171(8):729–735, 2006

Glass N, Dearwater S, Campbell JC: Intimate partner violence screening and intervention: data from eleven community hospital emergency departments in Pennsylvania and California. J Emerg Nurs 27(2):141–149, 2001 11275861

HEAL Trafficking: HEAL Trafficking and Hope for Justice's protocol toolkit for developing a response to victims of human trafficking in health care settings. 2019. Available at: https://healtrafficking.org/protocol-toolkit-for-developing-a-response-to-victims-of-human-trafficking-in-health-care-settings. Accessed November 8, 2019.

Iyengar R: Does the certainty of arrest reduce domestic violence? Evidence from mandatory and recommended arrest laws. Journal of Public Economics 93(1–2):85–98, 2009

Kentucky. Rev. Stat. Ann. § 209A.010 (West 2008)

Love H, Hussemann J, Yu L, et al: Justice in their own words: perceptions and experiences of (in)justice among human trafficking survivors. Urban Institute. March 2018. Available at: www.urban.org/sites/default/files/publication/97351/justice_in_their_own_words_0.pdf. Accessed November 9, 2019.

McDonald C: Cry Purple: One Woman's Journey Homelessness, Crack Addiction, and Prison to Blindness, Motherhood, and Happiness. Scotts Valley, CA, CreateSpace Independent Publishing Platform, 2013

McDonald C: The Same Kind of Human: Seeing the Marginalized and Exploited Through Eyes of Grace, Author, 2016

New Mexico Stat. Ann. § 27-7-14 to 21 (West 2008)

Office of Minority Health, U.S. Dept of Health and Health Services: National Standards for Culturally and Linguistically Appropriate Services (CLAS) in Health and Health. 2019. Available at: www.thinkculturalhealth. hhs.gov/assets/pdfs/EnhancedNationalCLASStandards.pdf. Accessed November 8, 2019.

Rodríguez MA, McLoughlin E, Campbell JC: Mandatory reporting of domestic violence injuries to the police: what do emergency department patients think? JAMA 286(5):580–583, 2001 11476660

Rodríguez MA, Sheldon WR, Rao N: Abused patient's attitudes about mandatory reporting of Intimate partner abuse injuries to police. Women Health 35(2–3):135–147, 2002 12201504

Shandro J, Chisolm-Straker M, Duber HC, et al: Human trafficking: a guide to identification and approach for the emergency physician. Ann Emerg Med 68(4):501–508, 2016 27130802

Smith HA: Walking Prey: How America's Youth are Vulnerable to Sex Slavery. New York, Palgrave Macmillan, 2014, p 123

Smith HA: Walking Prey: How America's Youth are Vulnerable to Sex Slavery. New York, Palgrave Macmillan, 2014, p 37

State of Nevada, NRS 629.041, Provider of Health Care to Report Persons Having Injuries Apparently Inflicted by Knife or Firearm in Non-accidental Circumstances. 1977. Available at: www.leg.state.nv.us/nrs/nrs-629.html#NRS629Sec041. Accessed November 8, 2019.

State of Nevada, NRS 629.045, Provider of health care to report persons having certain burns; immunity of certain persons from civil action for disclosure. 1991. Available at: www.leg.state.nv.us/nrs/nrs-629.html#NRS629Sec045. Accessed November 8, 2019.

Stratton K, Shetty P, Wallace R, et al. (eds): Institute of Medicine Committee to Assess the Science Base for Tobacco Harm Reduction. Washington, DC, National Academies Press, 2001

Trafficking Victims Protection Act of 2000, Pub. L. No. 106-386

U.S. Department of State: Rights and protections for temporary workers. U.S. Visas, 2019. Available at: https://travel.state.gov/content/travel/en/us-visas/visa-information-resources/temporary-workers.html. Accessed November 9, 2019.

Victims of Trafficking and Violence Protection Act of 2000, Pub. L. No. 106-386

Young Women's Empowerment Project: Girls do what they have to do to survive: illuminating methods used by girls in the sex trade and street economy to fight back and heal. 2009. Available at: https://ywepchicago.files.wordpress.com/2011/06/girls-do-what-they-have-to-do-to-survive-a-study-of-resilience-and-resistance.pdf. Accessed November 9, 2019.

Index

Page numbers printed in **boldface** *type refer to tables or figures.*

Acceptance and commitment therapy, 87
Accommodation, and access to health care, 177, **178**
Action-Means-Purpose (A-M-P) model, **226**
Addiction and Trauma Recovery Model (ATRIUM), 140
Adolescents, as trafficked persons. *See also* Children
common medical conditions in, 83–86
health care coverage for, 93
identification of in health care system, 57–58
interviewing of, 239
mental health care for, 87–88
Advocacy, by clinicians, 10–11, 213–214, 218–220
Aftercare services, and psychotherapy for trafficked persons, 162
Agenda for Sustainable Development (United Nations), 22
Amaya, Barbara, 228–229
American Academy of Family Physicians, 6
American Bar Association, 220
American Hospital Association, 6
American Medical Association, 6
American Medical Women's Association, 6
American Psychological Association, 6

American Public Health Association, 6, 31
And Life Continues: Sex Trafficking and My Journey to Freedom (Barnes 2015), 234
Anxiety, in trafficked children, 175
Arizona, and mandated reporting, 228
Assessment. *See also* Diagnosis; Screening
definition of, **34**
disclosure of results, 40–41
general principles of, 35–36
sensitivity and specificity of structured measures, 39–40
special populations and, 41–42
of substance use disorders, 139
validation of tools for, 36–39
Attachment, and psychotherapy, **151**
Authorization, for use of protected health information, 215–216, 218–220

Barnes, Wendy, 233–234
Behavior. *See also* Cognitive behavioral therapy
discomfort of health care professionals with trafficked persons, 56
traumatic response in trafficked persons and, 73–74

Bias, and treatment of trafficked
persons with substance use disorders, 142–144
Biopsychosocial model, and mental
health services for trafficked
persons, 200, **201**
Blue Campaign (Homeland Security), 126
Borderline personality disorder,
144
Brain, effects of trauma on development, 141
Brochures, on services available to
trafficked persons, 125
Bucceroni, Greg, 238–239
Buddhism, and mental health care
for trafficked persons, 181

Case examples
of criminal activity by trafficked
person, 65
of labor trafficking, 19, 31,
49–50, 119, 229–232,
234–237, 240–241, 244–245
of sex trafficking, 79, 91, 152,
169, 174, 226–228, 233–234,
238–239, 242–243, 246–248
of substance use disorder, 133
Case management, and integrated
care approach, 99
Category fallacy, and cultural context of mental health issues,
197
C-Change program (West Coast
Children's Clinic), 181
Center for Integrated Health Solutions, 100
Centers for Disease Control and
Prevention, 97, 125
Centers for Medicare and Medicaid
Services, 214
Child abuse
case example of, 237–238
reporting requirements for, 218,
237

as risk factor for trafficking, 3, **4,**
172
Child Abuse Prevention and Treatment Act (2016), 40, 72,
227–228, 237
Children, as trafficked persons.
See also Adolescents; Child
abuse; Child sex trafficking;
Special populations
common medical conditions in,
83–86
effects of trauma on brain development, 141
health needs of, 174–176
identification of in health care
system, 57–58
labor trafficking and, 170
mental health therapy for,
180–182, **183–184**
Child sex trafficking (CST)
case example of, 169, 174
definition of human trafficking
and, 171, 169–171
epidemiology of, 171–174
health care access and, 176–180
mental health therapy and,
180–182, **183–184**
study of children at risk for, 24
Child Welfare Information Gateway, 125, 127
Christine's Vision, 244
Chronic disease, management of,
98
Clinicians. *See also* Advocacy;
Health care professionals;
Mental health care
competence in psychotherapy for
trafficked persons, **157,**
160–162
cultural competence of, 199
disclosure of patient status and
HIPAA, 214–218
training in mental health therapy for trafficked children,
183

Clinton Global Initiative, 237, 249

Coalition to Abolish Slavery and Trafficking, 236–237

Coercion techniques, of traffickers, 5–6

Cognitive-behavioral therapy (CBT), 202

Cognitive processing therapy, 140, 161

Collaboration, and trauma-informed approach to health care, 121

Collaborative/integrated approach, to integration of primary and mental health care, 99, 100

Colocated model, of integrated primary and mental health care, 99, 100

CommonSpirit Health, 123, 234

Communication, and cultural issues in mental health care for trafficked persons, 197–198. *See also* Language

Community interventions, and mental health care for trafficked persons, 203–204

Comorbidity, of trauma and substance use in trafficked persons, 140

Complex presentations, and encounters of health care professionals with trafficked patients, 56–57

Concept map, of life cycle of exploitation, **25**

Confidentiality, for trafficked persons in health care settings, 69, 71, 72, 124. *See also* Health Insurance Portability and Accountability Act of 1996

Congo, and mental health care for trafficked persons, 181

Consultative/coordinated approach, to integrated primary and mental health care, 99–100

Convergent Functional Information for Suicidality Scale (CFI-S), 38

Coping skills, and psychotherapy for trafficked persons, 154, 155

Countertransference, and treatment of trafficked persons with substance use disorders, 142–144

Covenant House, 171

"Covered entity," under HIPAA, 214

Criminal activity, and case example of human trafficking, 65

Criminal justice system. *See* Law enforcement

Crisis, and public health, 6–7, 12

Crisis stabilization, and psychotherapy for trafficked persons, 155

Cry Purple (McDonald 2013), 243

CUES Intervention, 123

Culture, and cultural issues. *See also* Language

cultural competence of mental health professionals, 199

culturally informed interventions for mental health issues in trafficked persons, 200–205

diagnosis and treatment of mental health issues in trafficked persons, 196–200

importance of in working with trafficked persons, 195–196, 230, 231

mental health therapy for trafficked children and, 184

traditional healers and mental health care for trafficked persons, 181–182

trafficking of children and, **173**, 174, 179

trauma-informed approach to health care and, 121

treatment of substance abuse disorders and, 142

Dance/movement therapy, 184
Decision making
  disclosure of patient information
    and, **222**
  selection of psychosocial inter-
    ventions and, 204–205
Dental injuries, in trafficked persons, 82–83
Department of Human Services, 216
Depression
  psychotherapy for trafficked per-
    sons and, 154
  trafficking of children and, 175
Diagnosis. *See also* Assessment
  mental health care for trafficked
    persons and, 196–200
  misdiagnosis of human traffick-
    ing in health care setting,
    50–51
Dignity Health, 123–124, 125, 225,
  232, 248
Documentation, and case example
  of sex trafficking, 227
Domestic violence
  mandated reporting on, 245–246
  as public health problem, 23
  resources on risk factors and in-
    dicators for, 125
  response to in health care sys-
    tem, 53
  screening for, 126
DSM-5 (American Psychiatric Association 2013), 134, 200

Economics. *See* Poverty; Profits;
  Socioeconomic barriers; Sustainable development
Education. *See also* Psychoeducation; Schools; Training
  on mental health care for traf-
    ficked children, 183
  on patient-centered and trauma-
    informed care, 43, 74,
    121–123, 123–124
  on sex trafficking, 248

Elder abuse, 127
*Elder Abuse Screening Tools for
  Healthcare Professionals*
  (National Center on Elder
  Abuse 2016), 127
Eleven Inc., 125
Emergency department. *See also*
  Health care system
  addressing health effects of hu-
    man trafficking in, 67, 69
  case example of sex trafficking
    and, 229
  encounters with and identifica-
    tion of trafficked persons in,
    66–67
  health effects of human traffick-
    ing in, **70**
  mandated reporting and, 72
  obligations under Medicare and
    Medicaid, 240
  patient history and physical ex-
    ams in, 69, 71–72
  referrals for additional re-
    sources, 74, 236
  trauma-informed care and,
    72–74
Emergency Medical Treatment and
  Active Labor Act (1985), 240
Emotional reactions, and psychotherapy for trafficked persons,
  154
Empowerment
  mental health therapy for traf-
    ficked children and, 184
  psychotherapy for trafficked per-
    sons and, 162
  trauma-informed care and, 73,
    121
Epidemiology, of human trafficking,
  22–26, 171–174. *See also*
  Prevalence
Exposure therapy, 161
Eye movement desensitization and
  reprocessing (EMDR), 202, 203
Eyes Open International, 241

FACT SHEET: Human Trafficking (Administration for Children and Families 2017), 126

Family. *See also* Parents
mental health care for trafficked persons and, 204
rejection of trafficked persons by, 157

Federal Bureau of Investigation, 125

Federally Qualified Health Centers, **94**

Fishing industry, and labor trafficking, 175, 176

Food insecurity, and cost as barrier to health care, 93–94. *See also* Malnutrition

Forced migrants, 195, 196. *See also* Undocumented immigrants

Forensic documentation, 227

Forensic sexual assault exam, 82

Freud, Sigmund, 143

Futures Without Violence, 123, 125

Gender. *See also* Transgendered individuals
cultural issues in mental health care for trafficked persons, 199, 200
demographics of sex trafficking and, 55

Genitourinary exam, in emergency department, 71, 72

Global Slavery Index, 2, 21

Gold standard, for validation of screening tools and assessment measures, 37, **38**, 40

Gould, Tanya, 248

Group therapy, 162, 204

Guanzon, Angela, 244–245

Harm reduction model, and health care for trafficked persons, 10, 23, 233

HEAL Trafficking, 44, 123–124, 127, 245

Health. *See also* Health care system; Mental health; Public health
common conditions in trafficked persons, 80–86
consequences of human trafficking, 7, 50, 67, 69, **70**, 92
labor exploitation and occupational, 22
needs of trafficked children, 174–176

Health care professionals (HCPs). *See also* Health care system
identification of trafficked persons by, 50
lack of awareness and knowledge about human trafficking, 53–55
role of in combating human trafficking, 10–11

Health care system. *See also* Emergency department; Health; Health care professionals; Mental health care; Patient-centered care, and patient-centered, survivor-centered approach; Trauma-informed care
access to and coverage for trafficked persons, 92–95
barriers to care for trafficked persons, 83, 85–86
child sex trafficking and access to, 176–180
chronic disease management and, 98
community health centers and, **94**
constraints on time and privacy in, 53–54
human trafficking response protocols and, 42–43
integration of primary and behavioral health care, 99
lack of trauma-informed, human trafficking-specialized practitioners, 53

Health care system (*continued*)
   language and access to, 95–96
   legal considerations for, 100–101
   misdiagnosis of human traffick-
      ing in, 50–51
   provider barriers to identifica-
      tion of trafficked persons in,
      54–57
   reproductive health and, 98–99
   safety planning for patients and,
      96–97
   screening and disease preven-
      tion in, 98
   self-identification of trafficked
      persons in, 57
   special populations as trafficked
      persons in, 57–58, 101–102
   substance use disorders and, 100
   system barriers to identification
      of trafficked persons in, 51–54
   trauma-informed approach to
      trafficked persons in, 96,
      120–121
   vaccines and, 97
Health insurance, and barriers to
   accessing health care, 93–94
Health Insurance Portability and
   Accountability Act of 1996
   (HIPAA), 74, 214–218, 228
Health Resources and Services
   Administration, 94, 100
*Help for Victims of Trafficking in
   Persons* (FBI 2019), 125
Hepatitis A and hepatitis B vac-
   cines, 97
Heroin, and substance use by traf-
   ficked persons, 138
HIPAA. *See* Health Insurance Por-
   tability and Accountability Act
   of 1996
HIV/AIDS
   child sex trafficking and, 175
   global estimates of, 21
   in trafficked adolescent males,
      85

Homeland Security, 126, 231
Homelessness, and housing
   health care coverage and re-
      quirement of residential
      address, 93
   patient safety and availability of
      shelter, 236
   as risk factor for human traffick-
      ing, 3, **4**
   risk of medical conditions in traf-
      ficked persons and, 82
Human papillomavirus (HPV) vaccine, 97
Human rights, public health and
   protection of, 20
Human trafficking. *See also*
   Advocacy; Assessment;
   Case examples; Culture;
   Health care system; Labor
   trafficking; Mental health care;
   Risk factors; Sex trafficking;
   Trafficked persons
   definitions of, 1, 20–22, **33,** 91,
      169–170
   epidemiology, consequences, and
      range of, 22–26
   myths and misconceptions
      about, **9,** 55–56
   patient-centered care and,
      42–44
   as public health issue, 6–8, 12
   role of health care professionals
      in combating, 10–11
   screening for, 32, 34–35, 37–42
Human Trafficking Identification
   Assessment Measure-14, 36–37
*Human Trafficking: Information
   for Health Care Providers*
   (Administration for Children
   and Families 2019), 126
*Human Trafficking 101: Dispelling
   the Myths* (Dignity Health),
   248
Hurt, Insult, Threaten, and Scream
   Tool (HITS), 126–127

ICD-10 (World Health Organization 1993), 200, 227
Identifiable Me, 248
Identity, reestablishment of cultural, 199
Idioms of distress, and cultural issues, 197, 198–199
Immigration. *See also* Undocumented immigrants
  resources for trafficked persons and, 159
  as risk factor for human trafficking, 3
  stages in process of, 195–196
"Improving the Quality of Health Care for Mental and Substance Use Conditions" (Institute of Medicine 2005), 99
Information resources. *See* National Human Trafficking Hotline; Referrals; Websites
Institute of Medicine, 99
Integrated care approach, for behavioral health and primary care, 87, 99
Integrated cognitive-behavioral therapy, 140
Intellectual developmental disorder (IDD), 41–42
International Labour Organization, 21, 66
Interpreters. *See* Language
Interviewing, of youth and young adults, 239. *See also* Motivational interviewing
Intimate Partner Violence and Sexual Violence Victimization Assessment Instruments for Use in Healthcare Settings (Centers for Disease Control and Prevention 2007), 127

Juju practices, and Nigerian culture, 180

Labor trafficking. *See also* Human trafficking; Trafficked persons
  case examples of, 19, 31, 49–50, 119, 229–232, 234–237, 240–241, 244–245
  children and, 170
  common medical conditions and, **81**
  demographics of compared to sex trafficking, 171–172
  frequency of compared to sex trafficking, 21, 66
  indicators of in emergency department, **68**
  occupational health and, 22
  screening tools for, 38
  spectrum of, **27**
  undocumented immigrants and, 241–242
  wage theft and, 26, **27**
  work-related trauma and illness associated with, 175–176
Language
  access to health care and, 95–96
  communication with trafficked persons and, 235
  cultural issues in mental health care for trafficked persons, 197–198, 200, 202
  emergency department and, 71
  as risk factor for human trafficking, 3, **4**
  screening tools and, 38
Law enforcement. *See also* Criminal activity; Legal issues
  arrests of trafficked persons for prostitution, 155, 157
  definition of human trafficking as crime, 21, 91
  forensic sexual assault exam, 82
  HIPAA and disclosure of protected health information, 215

Law enforcement (*continued*)
  psychoeducation on human traf-
    ficking, 157
  referrals to from emergency de-
    partment, 74
Legal issues. *See also* Law enforce-
    ment; Safe harbor laws
  authorization by trafficked per-
    son for release of informa-
    tion, 220
  care of trafficked persons in
    health care settings and,
    100–101
  state laws on mandated report-
    ing, 40–41, 216–218,
    232–233, 245–246
Life cycle, of exploitation, **25**
Logical standard, for screening
    tools and structured assess-
    ments, 37, **38**, 40
*Look Beneath the Surface: Child
  Exploitation Brochure*
  (Administration for Children
  and Families 2019), 126
*Look Beneath the Surface:
  Health Care Brochure*
  (Administration for Children
  and Families 2019), 126
*Look Beneath the Surface: Social
  Services Brochure* (Adminis-
  tration for Children and
  Families 2019), 126

Malnutrition, in trafficked persons,
    82, 84. *See also* Food insecu-
    rity; Nutrition
Mandated reporting
  of child abuse, 58, 237
  child sex trafficking and, 171,
    227–228
  of domestic violence, 245–246
  emergency department and, 72, 74
  of labor or sex trafficking of mi-
    nors, 40–41
  limits of confidentiality and, 124

state laws on, 40–41, 216–218,
    232–233, 245–246
Massachusetts, and health care
    coverage, 93
McDonald, Christine, 243
Media, and extent of human traf-
    ficking, 23
Medicaid, and health care coverage,
    92–93
Medical Assessment Tool, 160
Medication-assisted treatments, for
    substance abuse disorders, 140–
    141. *See also* Pharmacotherapy
Meditation, 182
Mental disorders. *See also* Depres-
    sion; Mental health; Mental
    health care; Personality disor-
    ders; Posttraumatic stress
    disorder; Special populations;
    Substance use disorders
  barriers to identification of traf-
    ficked persons in health care
    system and, 58
  bias among clinicians toward pa-
    tients with history of, 56
  screening tools and assessment
    measures for patients with,
    41–42
Mental health. *See also*
    Anxiety; Mental disorders;
    Mental health care
  consequences of human traffick-
    ing, 7, 50, 69
  immigration as risk factor for,
    196
  risk of being trafficked and, 41
Mental health care. *See also*
    Mental health; Patient-
    centered care, and patient-
    centered, survivor-centered
    approach; Psychosocial inter-
    ventions; Psychotherapy;
    Trauma informed care
  cultural issues in care for traf-
    ficked persons, 196–200

integration of with primary health care, 87, 99

role of providers in addressing medical needs, 86–87

special considerations for trafficked adolescents, 87–88

therapy for trafficked children, **178**, 180–182, **183–184**

Mental status examination (MSE), 198

Mindfulness practices, 182

Motivational interviewing, 155, 203

Multidisciplinary approach, to screening and assessment, **34**

Multifinality, and psychotherapy for trafficked persons, 154

Music therapy, 184

Myths and misconceptions, about human trafficking, **9**, 55–56

Narrative exposure therapy (NET), 161, 202

National Adult Protective Services Association, 125

National Domestic Violence Hotline, 125

National Human Trafficking Hotline, 74, 86, 97, 125, 127, 216, 217, 219, 220, 221, 234

National Human Trafficking Training and Technical Assistance Center (NHTTAC), 35

National Runaway Safeline, 125, 239

National Standards for Culturally and Linguistically Appropriate Services in Health and Health Care (U.S. Department of Health and Human Services), 95

National Survivor Network, 125, 236–237, 245

Natural disasters, as risk factor for child trafficking, **173**, 174

NEJM Catalyst (journal), 119–120

Nevada, and mandated reporting, 233

Nigeria, and cultural practices, 180

Nobody's Girl: A Memoir of Lost Innocence, Modern Day Slavery, and Transformation (Amaya 2015), 228–229

Nonmaleficence, bioethical principle of, 52

Nutrition, and medical conditions in trafficked persons, 82–83. *See also* Food insecurity; Malnutrition

Obama, Barack, 237, 249

Office on Trafficking in Persons, 126

Office for Victims of Crime, 124

Opioids, and substance use by trafficked persons, 138

Pacific Survivor Center, 123–124

Parents, and access to medical records of minors, 216. *See also* Family

Patient-centered care, and patient-centered, survivor-centered approach

definition of, **34**

PEARR tool and, 123–128

principles of trauma-informed approach and, 120–121

systematic screening or assessment for human trafficking and, 42–43

universal education and, 121–123

Patient-provider relationship, in emergency department, 69, 71. *See also* Therapeutic relationship

PEARR Tool, 123–128, 225–226, 232, 233

Peer support, and trauma-informed approach to health care, 121

Personality disorders, and substance use disorders, 144
Pharmacotherapy, and cultural issues, 203. *See also* Medication-assisted treatments; Prescription medications
Physical exams, in emergency department, 71–72
Pocket cards, for patient information about resources, 127
Posttraumatic stress disorder (PTSD)
   psychotherapy for trafficked persons and, 154, 161
   in trafficked children, 175, 176
Poverty, as social determinant of child trafficking, 172
Prescription medications, access to by trafficked persons, 98
Pregnancy, and medical complications in trafficked adolescents, 85
Prevalence. *See also* Epidemiology
   estimates of for human trafficking, 171
   of substance use disorders in trafficked persons, 134–138
Privacy, in health care settings, 53–54, 69, 71
Profits, of human trafficking, 8, 23
Prostitutes and prostitution, and legal issues in sex trafficking, 55, 155, 157
"Protected health information," and HIPAA, 214–215
Protocols
   definition of, **34**
   for human trafficking response in health care institutions and professional organizations, 43–44
Psychoeducation
   for law enforcement agencies, 157
   mental health therapy for trafficked children and, 184

Psychological consequences, of human trafficking, 7–8, **151,** 153–155
Psychosocial interventions, and cultural issues in mental health care, 202–203, 204–205
Psychotherapy, for trafficked persons. *See also* Acceptance and commitment therapy; Cognitive behavioral therapy; Cognitive processing therapy; Group therapy; Mindfulness practices
   extra-individual factors in, 155–162, 163
   intra-individual factors in, 150–155, 162–163
Public health. *See also* Health care system
   domestic violence and, 23
   human trafficking as issue in, 6–8, 12
   protection of human rights as essential to, 20
   trauma-informed care and, 122
Push and pull factors, and risk for human trafficking, 3–6

Quick Youth Indicators for Trafficking (QYIT), 35

Rape, Abuse and Incest National Network, 125
Recidivism, and survivors of trafficking, 7–8
Recruitment methods, for child trafficking, 174
Red flags. *See also* Risk factors
   in case example of labor trafficking, 244–245
   in case example of sex trafficking, 227
   for identification of trafficking victims, 11
   for retention in treatment for substance abuse, 141–142

Referrals. *See also* Websites
emergency department and, 74
patient-centered care and,
127–128
Reintegration, of trafficked persons, 158–159
Reliability, of screening tools, 40
Religion, and mental health care for trafficked children, 180, 184
Reproductive health issues, in trafficked persons, 84–85, 98–99
Resilience, cultural themes of, 204
Revictimization, risk of for trafficked persons, 150
Risk factors, for human trafficking, 3–6, 172, **173**, 174, 247
Runaway status, as risk factor for human trafficking, 3, **4**

Safe harbor laws, 93, 100, 220
Safety, for trafficked persons as patients
mandated reporting on domestic violence and, 246
mental health therapy for trafficked children and, 184
planning considerations for health care systems and, 96–97
referrals from emergency department for additional resources, 74
safety cards or brochures with information on resources, 125
trauma-informed approach to health care and, 121
Same Kind of Human: Seeing the Marginalized and Exploited Through Eyes of Grace (McDonald 2016), 243
Schools, and health care services, 93
Screening, and screening tools. *See also* Assessment
definition of, **33**
disease prevention and, 98
disclosure of results, 40–41
general principles of, 32, 34–35
recommendations of U.S. Preventive Services Task Force (USPSTF), **107–118**
sensitivity and specificity of, 39–40
special populations and, 41–42
treatment for trafficked persons and, 160
validation of tools for, 37–39, 53
Screening Tool for Victims of Human Trafficking, 160
Seeking Safety, 149
Self-esteem, and psychotherapy for trafficked persons, 154
Self-identification, of trafficked persons, 67
Sensitivity, of screening tools and assessment measures, **34**, 39–40
Sexual abuse
as risk factor for sex trafficking, 3, **4**, 172, 247
state reporting requirements and definition of, 218
Sex trafficking. *See also* Child sex trafficking; Human trafficking; Trafficked persons
case examples of, 79, 91, 152, 169, 174, 226–228, 233–234, 238–239, 242–243, 246–248
common medical conditions and, **81**
definition of, 20–21
indicators of in emergency department, **68**
misconceptions and stereotypes about, 55
screening tools for, 38
Short Screen for Child Sex Trafficking (SSCST), 35, 39, 40
Skin exam, in emergency department, 71, 72
Slavery, and human rights, 20

Social justice, and mental health therapy for trafficked children, 184

Social networks, and cultural issues in mental health care, 203. *See also* Supportive networks

Social workers, 219, 240

Socioeconomic barriers, to psychotherapy for trafficked persons, **156**, 158–159

Special populations. *See also* Adolescents; Children; Mental disorders

    barriers to identification of as trafficked persons in health care system, 57–58

    screening tools and assessment measures for identification of as trafficked persons, 41–42

    special considerations for in health care system, 101–102

Specificity, of screening tools and assessment measures, **34**, 39–40

States. *See also* Legal issues; Safe harbor laws; *specific state*

    Medicaid programs and, 92–93

    variation in laws on mandated reporting, 40–41, 216–218, 232–233, 245–246

Stereotypes, about trafficked persons in health care system, 55

Stigma

    psychotherapy for trafficked persons and, 155, **156**, 157

    treatment of trafficked persons with substance use disorders, 142–144

Substance use disorders, in trafficked persons

    assessment of, 139

    bias of clinicians toward patients with history of, 56

    case example of, 133–134

    children and, 175

    health care system and assessment of patients for, 100

    prevalence of, 134–138

    sex trafficking and, 243

    treatment for, 138, 139–144

Suicide, and suicidal ideation, 7, 175

Supportive networks, and psychotherapy for trafficked persons, **156**, 157–158. *See also* Social networks

Survivor, use of term, 12, **33**

Sustainable development, and United Nations, 22

Tai chi, and mental health care for trafficked children, 182

Tatoos, as indication of human trafficking, 232

Td/Tdap vaccines, 97

Texas, and study of children at risk for sexual exploitation, 24

Therapeutic alliance, and psychotherapy for trafficked persons, 161

Therapeutic relationship, and motivational interviewing, 203. *See also* Patient-provider relationship

Town Watch Integrated Services, 239

Traditional healers, and mental health care for trafficked children, 181–182, 184

Trafficked persons. *See also* Adolescents; Children; Culture; Health; Health care system; Human trafficking; Mental health; Mental health care; Special populations; Substance use disorders

    definition of, **33**

    diversity of, 2–3

estimated numbers of, 1–2
identification of, 36, **52,** 53–59,
66–67
physical and psychological consequences for, 7–8
Trafficking Victim Identification
Tool (TVIT), 36
Trafficking Victims Protection Act
of 2000 (TVPA), 1, 20–21,
100–101, 225, **226,** 231
Training, in recognition of trafficked persons by health care
professionals, 11. *See also*
Education
Transgendered individuals, and
barriers to health care, 85.
See also Gender
Trauma. *See also* Trauma-informed
care
behaviors and response to in
trafficked persons, 73–74
effects of on brain, 141
history of and mental health
care for trafficked persons,
198
trafficked children and, 176
trauma bonding and, 5–6, 8, 179
Trauma, Addiction, Mental Health,
and Recovery (TAMAR), 140
Trauma Affect Regulation Guide
for Education and Therapy
(TARGET), 140, 181
Trauma-informed care
advocacy and authorization for
release of information, 219
definition of, **34**
emergency department and,
72–74
medical interpreters and, 95
principles of, 120–121
sexual abuse and, 237–238
for trafficked children, 184
training and education in for
health care professionals,
11, 43

Trauma and Recovery (Herman
1992), 196
Trauma Recovery and Empower-
ment Model (TREM), 140
Treatment plans, and psychother-
apy for trafficked persons, 162
Trust, and psychotherapy, 150, **151,**
152–153
T visa program, 159
TVPA. *See also* Trafficking Victims
Protection Act of 2000

*Uncovering the Truth: Identifying
Sexually Exploited Youth in a
Health Setting* (video), 239
Undocumented immigrants. *See
also* Immigration
health care services for, 93
labor trafficking and, 241–242
Trafficking Victims Protection
Act of 2000 and, 100–101
United Nations, 1, 20, 22, 169–170
U.S. Advisory Council on Human
Trafficking, 241
U.S. Department of Labor, 236
U.S. Department of State, 235
U.S. Human Trafficking Reporting
System, 171
U.S. Preventive Services Task Force
(USPSTF), 98, **107–118,** 126
Universal Declaration of Human
Rights, 20

Vacatur laws, 220
Vaccines, for trafficked persons, 97
Validation, of screening tools and
assessment measures, **34,**
36–39
Victims, use of term, 12, **33,** 170
Violence and Human Trafficking
Prevention and Response Pro-
gram (CommonSpirit Health),
234
Vulnerability factors, for child traf-
ficking, **173**

Wage theft, and labor abuse,
26, **27**
Websites, and information resources on health care and
mental health care for trafficked persons, 94, 97, 100, 126,
127, 128, 220, 228, 229, 232,
234, 235, 239, 241, 244, 248
West Coast Children's Clinic,
181

"What to Look for in a Health Care
Setting" (National Human
Trafficking Hotline 2016), 125
White House Advisory Council on
Human Trafficking, 232, 248
World Health Organization, 21,
203–204. *See also* ICD-10

Yoga, and mental health care for
trafficked children, 182